High Blood Pressure and You

The Effects of High Blood Pressure, Prescription Medication Side Effects, and Natural Ways To Reduce and Control High Blood Pressure

Clyde Verhine

ISBN: 1542592666

ISBN-13: 978-1542592666

Table of Contents: *Page*

Clyde Verhine

Facts You Should Know And Questions to Ask About High Blood Pressure:

In America today, one in three adults have high blood pressure, and after age 60 over six in ten Americans have it.

It is estimated that of this large number of Americans that have high blood pressure, over 1 in 5 don't know it.

High blood pressure contributes to over 1000 deaths in the US every day.

Do you worry that you may have high blood pressure or may suffer from it in the future?

Do you know why high blood pressure is known as the "silent killer"?

Do you know what causes high blood pressure?

Have you been diagnosed with high blood pressure and given prescription medication to control it?

Do you know what the different types of prescription medication are and how they work?

If you take prescription medication, do you know the risks and potential side effects of the drug(s)?

Do you know that millions of Americans who have been diagnosed and put on medication still do not have their blood pressure under control?

Can you check your own blood pressure at home?

Do you know that treatment for high blood isn't limited to prescription drugs?

Do you know about any of the natural methods of lowering blood pressure with or without the use of prescribed medication?

Do you know what nutrients the body needs to maintain healthy blood pressure?

Do you know what foods contain these nutrients and ways to increase them in your diet?

Do you know the best exercises to do to reduce high blood pressure?

Do you think that supplements are a good alternative if your diet does not include enough healthy foods?

Do you know which supplements or combination of supplements may be toxic?

You can get the answers to all of these questions without this book if you want to spend the time it takes to go to multiple sources, each of which usually cover only one topic of the many different aspects of high blood pressure and blood pressure control. I spent many hours reading a large amount of books, magazine articles, published scientific papers, and internet sources looking for consensus from experts in the fields of science and medicine. My focus was to identify the factual information that is important, and discarding popular or commercial myths. I also included the things in this book that I personally tried with the successful result of lowering my blood pressure to the point that I no longer need prescription medication to control my blood pressure. The aim of this book is to give you this information in one place and to tie it together in a more concise and understandable way.

The CDC reports these facts about High Blood Pressure:

About 7 of 10 people having their first heart attack have high blood pressure.

About 8 of 10 people having their first stroke have high blood pressure.

Since 1 in 3 adults already have high blood pressure, and the older you are the greater the chance that you have or will have this potentially deadly condition, you need to take the action today.

From this book you will get a better understanding of the meaning and the different levels of high blood pressure, what causes it, who is at risk, and the consequences of having it. You will learn about the ways blood pressure is measured and methods to monitor your blood pressure at home. You will also learn about the different types of medication being prescribed today to lower high blood pressure and the potential side effects of each type. The **Natural Blood Pressure Control** chapter of this book will present natural methods you can use to effectively reduce and control high blood pressure. Following these methods has the potential to reduce and even eliminate the need for prescription medication and their associated costs and unwanted side effects.

CHAPTER 1 ---
WHY I WROTE THIS BOOK

"If you don't take care of your body, where are you going to live?" ~ Unknown

For several years during my annual checkups, my doctor would tell me that my blood pressure was borderline high and he wanted to write me a prescription for it. Since except for the blood pressure concern, my health was excellent, I resisted for several years thinking that if it did not get any worse, I would not need medication. Eventually a combination of a high stress in a long hours job as a manager in a corporate manufacturing company, a life style where too often it was coffee for breakfast, fast food for lunch, processed frozen foods or pizza for dinner, and little or no time to exercise took its toll. My blood pressure continued to rise so I relented and let my doctor write me a prescription. He gave me a prescription for an ACE inhibitor type blood pressure medication. It worked somewhat but after about a year, I was experiencing fluctuations in my pressure readings so my doctor gave me a second prescription for a beta-blocker type blood pressure medicine to take along with the ACE inhibitor medication.

My doctor never discussed in detail the possible side effects of these drugs or what would happen if I stopped taking them, and I did not ask about possible alternatives. About a year and a half ago, my doctor gave up his private practice to take a position at a university hospital. Before I selected a new doctor to go to for my annual checkup, my prescriptions had expired and I could get no more refills. I felt certain that I was experiencing some side effects caused by these two drugs and decided to stop taking them. I stopped taking the beta-blocker first and then after about a month I stopped taking the ACE inhibitor. Knowing what I know now after doing more in-depth research, I was lucky and did not experience the potentially severe consequence of stopping the beta-blocker medication without consulting a doctor (more about this will be discussed in the side effects chapter of this book).

I had a digital home blood pressure cuff that I had used occasionally to monitor my blood pressure. After stopping the medication, I used the cuff to check my pressure about two or three times a week to make sure it was staying under control. Then one day my blood pressure went up drastically and stayed above 155/104 for several days. Since I had still not visited a new doctor, I was very concerned about what was causing such a spike. Thinking about this I remembered that the night before the spike began that my wife and I had gone to a local Chinese buffet restaurant for dinner. I began to think that maybe the MSG or excessive salt in the food was responsible. This spike in my blood pressure made me begin more in-depth research on what causes high blood pressure, the medications used to treat it, and what non-prescription methods could be used to lower blood pressure. I used research methods I learned when I was a student at the University of Georgia. In this quest for knowledge, I spent many hours reading a large amount of books, magazine articles, published scientific papers, and internet sources looking for consensus from experts in the fields of science and medicine. I focused on identifying what was important and eliminating what was just popular myth.

I am not saying this will work for everyone, but in trying to get my blood pressure down and under control, I started making changes to my lifestyle by following some of the methods I will talk about in the "Natural Blood Pressure Control" chapters of this book. I set an initial target goal getting my pressure back to less than 140/90 and started checking my blood pressure several times a day. After a few weeks of following some of these methods, my pressure was back down to an average of 134/84. That was about the same as the readings I was getting during my visits to the doctor when I was still taking my prescriptions. I honestly expect these reading to get better and I now feel much better than I have in a long time. I am not experiencing the side effects of the prescriptions I was taking - feeling weak and tired, unable to spend much time in direct sunlight, insomnia, and chronic coughing. After seeing the results I had gotten, I decided to write this book because I knew that others would benefit from what I have learned. All of this information is available out there if you want to spend the time to go to multiple sources to cover all the different areas. The aim of this book is to present this information in one place and tie it together in a more concise and understandable way. This book is not intended to be a replacement for professional medical care. The purpose of this book is to be educational and is intended to give the reader a better understanding of the subject matter. By being more informed you can improve your health and if you are under a doctor's care can help your doctor help you.

"Cherish your health: If it is good, preserve it. If it is unstable, improve it. If it is beyond what you can improve, get help." ~ George Carlin in "How To Stay Young"

~~~~~~~~~~

CHAPTER 2 ---
UNDERSTANDING

From this book, you will get a better understanding of the meaning of high blood pressure, what causes it, who is at risk, and the consequences of having it. You will also learn about the different types of high blood pressure medication being prescribed today and the potential side effects of each type. The Natural Blood Pressure Control chapter of this book will present natural methods you can easily use to effectively reduce and control high blood pressure. Following these natural methods has the potential to eliminate the need for prescription medication and their associated side effects.

A: What Is Blood Pressure?

In order to live, your body needs the energy and oxygen supplied by your blood. When your heart beats, it pumps blood throughout your body. As the blood is pumped, it pushes against the sides of your blood vessels. Simply put the force of this pushing or how hard your blood is pushing against the walls of your blood vessels is your blood pressure. When your heart beats, it pumps and then rests. It is the ebb and flow of the blood pushed by your heart pumping then resting that is measured and called blood pressure. Blood pressure that is too low is called hypotension and pressure that is consistently too high is called hypertension. The focus of this book will be on high blood pressure and hypertension.

Blood pressure is usually measured and recorded using two numbers that are written as a ratio. The top number (systolic) is the pressure in the vessels when the heart contracts (pumps). The bottom number (diastolic) measures the pressure when the heart is filling between contractions (resting).

Blood pressure is usually measured with a sphygmomanometer. This device was introduced in 1896 by the Italian physician Scipione Riva-Rocc. The word sphygmomanometer was put together from the Greek word *sphygmos* which means the beating (pulse) of the heart and the word manometer which is a device for measuring pressure or tension. Historically these devices used the height of a column of mercury to measure blood pressure in millimeters of mercury (mm Hg). You will still see measurements reported this way even though modern aneroid and electronic devices used to measure blood pressure do not contain mercury.

Blood pressure naturally rises and falls depending on the time of day, physical exertion, and other factors. Several measurements averaged over the course of at least a day or even longer should be used to determine which stage of blood pressure you have. So what do the blood pressure measurement readings indicate?

Normal - 120/80 mm Hg is considered to be a normal blood pressure reading in a healthy adult younger than age 60.

High-Normal - (Pre-hypertension) is when the systolic (top number) reads between 121 and 140 and/or the diastolic (bottom number) reads between 81 and 90. If your pressure is in the pre-hypertension range, you should continue to monitor and take measures to reduce.

High blood pressure - (Stage 1 Hypertension) is when the systolic (top number) reads between 141 and 159 and/or the diastolic (bottom number) reads between 91 and 99. If you are a younger than 60 and have consistent readings in this range you should take steps to reduce it and seek professional medical advice. A 2013 report published online in the *Journal of the American Medical Association* said that adults 60 or older should only take blood pressure medication if their blood pressure exceeds 150/90. The report stated that there was no clinical evidence showing that stricter guidelines provided any additional benefit to the patients.

High blood pressure - (Stage 2 Hypertension) is when the systolic (top number) reads 160 or higher and/or the diastolic (bottom number) reads 100 or higher. At any age if you have consistent readings in this range you should seek professional medical advice.

High blood pressure - (Hypertensive Crisis) If your systolic reading is 180 or higher and/or your diastolic reading is 110 or higher, wait a couple of minutes and take it again. Hypertensive Crisis readings that remain at or above 180/110 more than a couple of minutes indicate the need for immediate medical care.

~~~~~~~~~~

B: What Causes High Blood Pressure?

In America today, one in three adults has high blood pressure, and after age 60, over six in ten Americans have it. High blood pressure contributes to over 1000 deaths in the US every day and it is estimated that one in five Americans who have high blood pressure do not know it.

Most medical references define high blood pressure as either primary hypertension or secondary hypertension. By far the highest number of cases fall into the primary hypertension category.

In most cases of primary hypertension, there is usually no one specific cause identifiable for high blood pressure. There are however several factors known to increase the risk. These include:

* Diet high in processed foods lacking needed vitamins and minerals

* High sodium (salt) consumption

* High refined sugar consumption

* Sedentary lifestyle

* Stress

* Being overweight

* Using tobacco

* Drinking too much alcohol

In most cases of secondary hypertension (consistent readings of 160/100 or higher) the cause is an underlying condition. This type of high blood pressure usually appears suddenly with readings that are usually higher than the readings from primary hypertension. Reasons that can cause secondary hypertension include:

* Chronic kidney disease

* Thyroid problems

* Sleep apnea

* Certain congenital blood vessel defects

* Excessive alcohol use and abuse

* Certain prescription and over the counter medications

* Illegal drugs such as cocaine, amphetamines, and others

* Pregnancy

In addition to the causes listed above, there are also some additional risk factors that may increase a person's chances for developing high blood pressure.

Potential risk factors for high blood pressure include:

* Age - As you get older, your chances greatly increase. After age 60, over 6 in 10 Americans have high blood pressure

* Race - African Americans have a higher risk for developing high blood pressure, and at an earlier age.

* Genetics - You have a greater chance of having high blood pressure if other close blood related members of your family have had it.

C: Symptoms & Measurement

Symptoms

If you think that you will just wait until you have some symptoms to check your blood pressure, you are taking a dangerous risk with your life. You can have high blood pressure with no obvious symptoms until you have a heart attack or stroke. There is a reason that high blood pressure is known as the "silent killer".

High blood pressure is usually a symptom-less condition and only displays symptoms when blood pressure spikes into a hypertensive crisis level. Remember a person is in hypertensive crisis if the systolic reading is 180 or higher and/or the diastolic reading is 110 or higher. This should be considered a medical emergency and the person should seek immediate medical attention. A hypertensive crisis can result in heart attack, stroke, or death. Some of the symptoms that may be present during a hypertensive crisis are severe headache, vision problems, fatigue, confusion, chest pain, difficulty breathing, difficulty speaking, nausea, fainting, and/or nosebleed.

There is only one way to know if you have high blood pressure. You either have to have a doctor or health professional measure it, or you have check it yourself with a blood pressure measuring device.

Measurement

High blood pressure cannot be diagnosed based on a single reading. Your doctor or heath care provider needs to take two or more readings during an appointment and then repeat the procedure again over several more medical appointments in order to properly diagnose that a patient has high blood pressure. Sometimes, a person's blood pressure reading will be higher in a doctor's or health care provider's office. This is called "white coat hypertension" and may be caused from the stress that can be associated with the medical appointment.

Since visiting a doctor to have your blood pressure checked on a daily basis would prove to be impractical and quite costly, it is recommended that you monitor blood pressure readings using a home blood pressure measuring device. Taking your own measurements will prove to be a powerful tool and allow you to take more control of your health. Seeing and measuring results will provide you an incentive to control your blood pressure, and gives you a method to track the results of changes you may be taking to lower it. Self-monitoring will also help detect "white coat hypertension".

The two main types of devices used to monitor blood pressure are either Aneroid (Manual) or Digital (Automatic).

Aneroid devices are considered more accurate and usually are the ones used to check blood pressure in a doctor's office. These type monitors have a cuff that wraps around a person's upper arm, a squeeze bulb used to inflate the cuff, a dial gauge with a pointer, and a stethoscope used to listen to your heart beat. While an aneroid device is normally cheaper than a digital device, they are more prone to damage, the bulb may be hard to squeeze especially if a person has arthritis, and since you have to listen to your heartbeat may present problems for those with hearing impairments. For these reasons, if you want to self-monitor your blood pressure at home or work, aneroid devices are usually not as practical as the digital models.

Digital models are usually battery operated, they inflate themselves, automatically take the readings, and display the reading on a digital screen. Since the digital models are simple to operate, require no special skill to use, and are less prone to damage, they are usually the choice made by those wanting to self-monitor their blood pressure. Digital models may either use a cuff that wraps around a person's upper arm or a wrist based cuff.

The most important features to look for when shopping for a home blood pressure cuff are accuracy, fit, and ease of use. Blood pressure cuffs are readily available for sale without a prescription at drug stores, some department stores, and some on-line shopping sites. Digital models with acceptable accuracy usually can be purchased for $50 to $90. These automatic digital models use either an upper arm cuff or a cuff that fits around your wrist. Proper fit is critical to the accuracy of these devices. If the cuff size is too small you will get a falsely high blood pressure reading, while if the cuff is too large you will get a falsely low blood pressure reading. The cuff size you need depends on your arm or wrist circumference. Since each manufacturer may use different specifications for cuff size (small, medium, large) be sure to check these specifications before deciding which size you should purchase. Ease of use should also be a very important factor in your purchase decision. The monitors should automatically inflate, have easy to read digital displays, and the control buttons should be easy to understand and operate. I personally prefer the wrist cuff type because it is more convenient. I don't have to have my upper arm bare in order to use it and it is a one-piece device that is smaller in size than an arm cuff model so it is easier to keep in a small case on my desk. Since it is faster and easier to use, I take and record readings more consistently.

While several brands currently have excellent online reviews, the brand that had the most consistent high reviews and recommendations has been Omron. Both their upper arm cuff monitors and their wrist cuff monitors have consistently received high reviews for accuracy, ease of use, and quality over the last several years. Regardless of the brand you purchase, be sure to follow the instructions for use for your specific device in order to get accurate readings.

Even those with normal blood pressure levels should self-monitor in order to be proactive in detecting any unusual blood pressure fluctuations and taking steps to correct or maintain a healthy level.

You should check your blood pressure at least twice a day and keep a record of the results. One feature of some of the newer digital blood pressure cuffs is a reading memory feature. I find it is easier to keep up with the averages by writing them down, but this is just a personal preference.

To check your pressure using a home blood pressure cuff:

* Relax and sit comfortably for 2 or 3 minutes with your legs uncrossed and with both feet on the floor.

* When you measure your blood pressure, be sure to follow your device's cuff and arm placement recommendations.

* Take three readings with at least 1 minute between each reading.

* Write down the average of these three readings and keep for your records.

For your two recorded readings per day, be sure to take one in the morning and one in the late afternoon at about the same times every day. To determine your true resting blood pressure you should not take a reading immediately after exercising or eating. Realize that your body has natural biological rhythms and your blood pressure will vary throughout the day. If you take a reading when you first get up in the morning, do not use that reading as your morning record. The body's normal circadian rhythm causes the adrenal glands to release serum cortisol when you first wake up. This can cause a significant increase in blood pressure. Because of this, people with very high blood pressure are most at risk for a heart attack or stroke in the morning hours. So wait 30 minutes to an hour after you get up before recording your morning reading

~~~~~~~~

D: Lowering Blood Pressure - What's In It For You?

What's in it for you? Recent studies show that high blood pressure may be the #1 cause of death factor in the world. Some of the risks involved with having high blood pressure include:

* Angina

* Coronary artery disease

* Damaged arteries

* Erectile dysfunction

* Hardened arteries

* Heart attack

* Heart damage

* Heart Failure

* Kidney disease

* Kidney failure

* Peripheral artery disease

* Stroke

* Vision loss

* Or Death

If you have high blood pressure now, you need to start immediately to get it back down to safe levels. If your pressure is in the normal range you should take actions and adopt habits that will help you keep and maintain it. The American Medical Association says that once damage is done to the heart, it cannot be undone by the body.

What's in it for you? Simply put, maintaining a healthy blood pressure is key to living a long and healthy life.

~~~~~~~~~~

CHAPTER 3 ---
PRESCRIPTION BLOOD PRESSURE MEDICATION

There are many types of drugs prescribed by doctors for the treatment of high blood pressure. Often a doctor will prescribe two or more different types of these drugs to be used in combination.

Although prescription drugs can save lives, they may also cause unwanted side effects. Since most drugs are ingested and absorbed in the digestive system, the most common side effects are nausea, constipation, dizziness, or diarrhea. While dizziness at first glance may not seem to be that serious, for elderly patients dizziness can cause a fall. Falls can lead to broken bones and a broken hip in an elderly person can take a deadly turn.

~~~~~~~~~~

A: Types Of Prescription Medications

When it comes to blood pressure medications, there are too many specific prescription trademarked drug names to list them all here, but most of them fall into the following generic categories:

* **Diuretics** - commonly called "water pills" that help the kidneys flush excess water and sodium by increasing urination. This drug, developed to treat high blood pressure in the 1950's, was the first drug prescribed for treating hypertension. Generic drug names include: amiloride hydrochloride, bumetanide, chlorothiazide, chlorthalidone, furosemide, hydrochlorothiazide, indapamide, metolazone, spironolactone, and triamterene.

* **Beta blockers** - these work directly on the heart by reducing the heart rate and force of pumping as well as relaxing arterial walls.

Generic drug names include: acebutolol, atenolol, betaxolol, bisoprolol fumarate, carteolol hydrochloride, metoprolol tartrate, metoprolol succinate, nadolol, penbutolol sulfate, pindolol, propranolol hydrochloride, solotol hydrochloride, and timolol maleate.

* **ACE inhibitors** (angiotensin-converting-enzyme) - these reduce the production of a hormone (angiotensin II) that causes blood vessels to narrow, especially in the kidneys. Generic drug names include: benazepril hydrochloride, captopril, enalapril, maleate, fosinopril sodium, lisinopril, moexipril, perindopril, quinapril hydrochloride, ramipril, and trandolapril.

* **ARBs** (angiotensin II receptor blockers) - these help relax blood vessels by blocking the effects of the hormone angiotensin II. Generic drug names include: candesartan, eprosartan mesylate, irbesarten, losartan potassium, telmisartan, valsartan, perindopril, quinapril hydrochloride, ramipril, and trandolapril.

* **CCBs** (calcium channel blockers) - these relax blood vessels by keeping calcium from entering heart and blood vessel cells. When calcium enters the smooth muscle cells of the heart and blood vessels, it causes a stronger and harder contraction. Some CCB's also slow the heart rate. Generic drug names include: amlodipine besylate, bepridil, diltiazem, hydrochloride, felodipine, isradipine, nicardipine, nifedipine, nisoldipine, and verapamil hydrochloride.

* **Alpha blockers** - these relax the muscle tone of the vessel walls by reducing nerve impulses to the blood vessels, allowing blood to flow more easily. Generic drug names include: doxazosin mesylate, prazosin hydrochloride, and terazosin hydrochloride.

* **Alpha-2 Receptor Agonist** - these decrease activity in the adrenaline-producing portion of the involuntary nervous system. Generic drug names include: methyldopa.

* **Alpha-Beta blockers** - these reduce nerve impulses to blood vessels and slow the heartbeat. Generic drug names include: carvedilol and labetalol hydrochloride.

* **Central Agonists** - these relax blood vessels by controlling nerve impulses to the vessels. Generic drug names include: alpha methyldopa, clonidine hydrochloride, guanabenz acetate, and guanfacine hydrochloride.

* **Peripheral adrenergic inhibitors** - these block neurotransmitters in the brain that keeps smooth muscles from constricting. Generic drug names include: guanadrel, guanethidine monosulfate, and reserpine.

* **Vasodilators** - these cause the muscles in the blood vessel walls to relax and causes the vessels to dilate (widen) which allows the blood to flow with less pressure. Generic drug names include: hydralazine hydrocholoride and minoxidil.

If you are taking a prescription blood pressure medication(s) that is not a generic brand and are not sure which type it is, just ask your pharmacist or doctor. The next chapter will take a more in-depth look at these different types of prescription blood pressure medications and the possible side effects that may be caused from drugs in each of these categories.

~~~~~~~~~

B: Side Effects

"First do no harm." ~ Hippocrates

When you are prescribed any drug, you should always ask your doctor and your pharmacist to tell you in detail about any potential side effects or possible interactions with other substances. The possible side effects from the most commonly prescribed blood pressure medications are listed below.

* Diuretics

Most diuretics make the kidneys release more sodium into your urine and by increasing urination. The sodium takes water from your blood which decreases the amount of fluid flowing through your blood vessels which in turn reduces the pressure on your vessel walls. Developed in the 1950's, diuretics were one of the first drugs used to treat hypertension.

Possible side effects:

- More frequent need to urinate
- Reduced levels of potassium in the blood
- Mineral loss
- Increased blood sugar levels
- Dehydration
- Dizziness
- Headaches
- Weakness
- Leg cramps
- Impotence
- Gout

* Beta blockers

Beta blockers lower blood pressure by acting directly on the heart. They work by reducing the heart rate, reducing the force of pumping, and relaxing arterial walls. Many of the side effects of beta blockers are directly related to the fact that beta blockers work by slowing the heart and that they also affect the respiratory system. Beta blockers should not be taken if you are considering pregnancy or if there is a chance of pregnancy. Beta blockers should not be withdrawn suddenly because of an increased risk for heart attack, other heart problems, or even death.

Possible side effects:

- Cold hands or feet

- Weakness

- Fatigue

- Dizziness

- Insomnia

- Impotence

- Depression

- Shortness of breath

- Difficulty breathing

- Weight gain

(Authors note: this was one of the two blood pressure medications I was taking (generic brand Metoprolol). As stated in the Why I Wrote This Book chapter, I stopped taking it without knowing the risks of that choice. In my research, I found that the FDA has issued a warning about this drug: "Warning: Don't stop taking metoprolol suddenly. If you do, you may experience worse chest pain, a jump in blood pressure, or even have a heart attack". This is why I continue to emphasize that you should know the potential side effect before you start taking any prescription medication and why natural methods of control are better.)

* ACE inhibitors (angiotensin-converting-enzyme)

ACE inhibitors reduce the production of angiotensin (a hormone) that causes blood vessels to narrow. Ace inhibitors are another medication that should not be taken if you are considering pregnancy or if there is a chance of pregnancy. They may be dangerous to both mother and baby during pregnancy and even result in the death of the newborn.

Possible side effects:

- Cough
- Fluid retention
- Skin rash
- Loss of taste
- High potassium levels
- Fetal abnormalities
- Fetal death

* ARBs (angiotensin II receptor blockers)

ARB's help relax blood vessels by blocking the effects of angiotensin II. It works by preventing angiotensin from binding to receptors on the blood vessel walls. ARB's also should not be taken if you are considering pregnancy or if there is a chance of pregnancy. They may be dangerous to the baby during pregnancy and even result in the death of the newborn.

Possible side effects:

- Dizziness
- Increased potassium levels
- Fatigue
- Muscle cramps
- Diarrhea
- Fetal death

* CCBs (calcium channel blockers)

CCB's relax blood vessels by keeping calcium from entering the smooth muscle cells of the heart and blood vessels. This decreases the strength and force of contractions in the heart and opens up narrowed blood vessels. Some also slow the heart rate. Use caution if you drink grapefruit juice because grapefruit juice interacts with some CCB's causing increased blood levels of the drug that increases the risk of side effects.

Possible side effects:

- Dizziness

- Constipation

- Headache

- Swollen ankles

- Fluid buildup in legs

- Flushing of face

- Heartburn

- Irregular heartbeat

* Alpha blockers

Alpha blockers relax the muscle tone of the vessel walls by reducing nerve impulses to the blood vessels. This dilates the vessels which allows blood to flow more easily. These drugs are also used to treat prostate enlargement.

Possible side effects:

- Dizziness

- Fainting

- Weakness

- Fast heart rate

- Nasal congestion

- Dry mouth

* Alpha-2 Receptor Agonist

Alpha-2 Receptor Agonist decrease activity in the adrenaline-producing portion of the involuntary nervous system. This type is often used for high blood pressure that develops during pregnancy because of infrequent adverse effects on the pregnant woman or the developing baby.

Possible side effects:

- Dizziness
- Drowsiness
- Headache
- Dry mouth
- Weakness

* Alpha-Beta blockers

Alpha-Beta blockers reduce nerve impulses to blood vessels and also slow the heartbeat. These are sometimes administered by intravenous (IV) injection to patients with severe high blood pressure. Doctors may also prescribe these to patients who have congestive heart failure. This type of drug may cause a sudden drop in blood pressure when you first get up in the morning or stand up suddenly. Abrupt withdrawal may trigger angina or a heart attack, or may even cause death.

Possible side effects:

- Dizziness
- Weakness
- Feeling faint
- Insomnia
- Depression
- Dry mouth
- Impotence

* Central Agonists

Central Argonists relax blood vessels by controlling nerve impulses to the vessels. These work similar to alpha-beta blockers in reducing blood pressure but follow a different nerve pathway. Similar to alpha-beta blockers, this type of drug also may cause a sudden drop in blood pressure when you first get up in the morning or stand up suddenly.

Possible side effects:

- Anemia

- Dizziness

- Weakness

- Feeling faint

- Constipation

- Drowsiness

- Impotence

- Dry Mouth

* Peripheral adrenergic inhibitors

Peripheral adrenergic inhibitors block neurotransmitters in the brain that keeps smooth muscles from constricting. Similar to others above, this type of drug may also cause a sudden drop in blood pressure when you first get up in the morning or stand up suddenly. It was one of the few hypertension drugs available in the 1950's. This type is rarely used today because of its numerous side effects and drug interactions.

Possible side effects:

- Diarrhea

- Dizziness

- Weakness

- Feeling faint

- Impotence

- Heartburn

- Indigestion

- Nasal congestion

- Insomnia

- Nightmares

- Depression

* Vasodilators

Vasodilators cause the muscles in the blood vessel walls to relax which causes the vessels to dilate (widen). This allows the blood to flow more easily. Because it interferes with the way vasodilators work, you should avoid drinking alcohol while taking these drugs. Vasodilators should not be taken if you are considering pregnancy, if there is a chance of pregnancy, if you are pregnant, or if you are breast feeding. Taking vasodilators other drugs may affect the way the drugs work or may increase the chance of side effects.

Possible side effects:

- Excessive hair growth

- Chest pain

- Fluid retention

- Irregular heartbeat

- Joint pain

- Swelling around the eyes

- Nausea

- Dizziness

- Headache

- Flushing

- Fetal abnormalities

What do I do if I take medication for high blood pressure and experience a side effect that really bothers me?

If your doctor prescribes medication for your high blood pressure be sure to ask about the drug up front before you begin the treatment. Be sure the doctor fully explains any potential side effects the drug may have and the consequences if you take the drug and then decide to stop. If you are taking prescription medication for high blood pressure and you are experiencing side effects that bother you, use the information you have learned and work with your doctor. Ask them what steps you can take to lessen or eliminate the unwanted side effects.

For some, side effects such as fatigue or diarrhea from prescription medication may subside with time. Ask your doctor if they can change the dosage or change to a different medication. Even better, ask your doctor about natural methods for reducing blood pressure. These methods will be discussed in later chapters of this book.

In some cases, your doctor may prescribe a combination of drugs to reduce your blood pressure and/or to reduce side effects. A word of caution, when first starting to take any new medication, be alert to any potential allergic reaction. Call 911 immediately if you develop swelling in your throat or face, vomiting, fainting, hives, or wheezing.

~~~~~~~~~~

CHAPTER 4 ---
NATURAL BLOOD PRESSURE CONTROL

"It is common sense to take a method and try it: If it fails, admit it frankly and try another. But above all, try something." ~ Franklin D. Roosevelt

Ultimately, you need to think of blood pressure control as a numbers game and realize that prescription medications are not the only solution for treating all health conditions. Lifestyle is an extremely important part in treating high blood pressure. If you can reduce your blood pressure by maintaining a healthy lifestyle, you might postpone, reduce, or even eliminate the need for prescription medication. One thing you must know and remember is that no one food, drink, supplement, or exercise is a magic wand by itself. The route to reducing and controlling high blood pressure is by living a healthy lifestyle.

Some simple lifestyle changes in the following areas may help you achieve the goal of maintaining healthy blood pressure levels:

Diet

Exercise

Stress Reduction

Things to Avoid

The importance of and ways to achieve these changes will be discussed in this chapter

~~~~~~~~~~

A: What To Eat

"Life expectancy would grow by leaps and bounds if green vegetables smelled as good as bacon." ~ Doug Larson

One of the most important factors in controlling blood pressure is having a healthy and balanced diet. To maintain, reduce, and control blood pressure you need to concentrate on items in your diet that will supply the minerals, vitamins, and other nutrients that are critical in blood pressure control. If your diet consists mainly of commercially made foods, you are probably not getting the proper levels of these vital nutrients.

If you want to maintain healthy blood pressure levels, what nutrients do the foods you eat need to have?

The Big 3:

Potassium, Magnesium, Calcium

Potassium, magnesium, and calcium are the most important minerals needed for good blood pressure management.

* **Potassium** helps balance out the negative effects of salt. It also plays an important role in many other body functions like various chemical reactions, nerve signal transmissions, fluid balance, and muscle contractions. Having a high salt/low potassium level reduces the ability of your kidneys to remove the excess salt.

* **Magnesium** increases the ability of the smooth muscle cells in the blood vessels to relax. Magnesium deficiency increases with age and it is estimated that as many of 75% of people in the United States have a magnesium deficiency. Healthy blood pressure levels depend on balanced ratios of magnesium to calcium.

***Calcium** helps blood vessels when they need to tighten and relax. Calcium not only helps blood vessels tighten and contract, it also aids the signal transmission in nerves and cells. If blood levels of calcium are low, your body will rob calcium from your bones to provide calcium to these functions.

Healthy blood pressure levels depend on balanced ratios of both Sodium to Potassium and Magnesium to Calcium. A healthy balanced diet is the best way to insure these ratios are maintained.

also important:

Coenzyme Q10 (CoQ10), Omega-3 fatty acids, Vitamin B-6, Vitamin C, and Vitamin D.

* **Coenzyme** Q10 is naturally made by the body and it functions like an antioxidant. Coenzymes also help enzymes speed up the rate of chemical reactions in cells.

* **Omega-3** fatty acids are considered essential fatty acids necessary for human health. Unlike CoQ10, Omega-3 fatty acids are not produced in the body, they can only be gotten through dietary sources.

* **Vitamin B-6** is naturally present in many foods. It helps control blood pressure by controlling homocysteine levels in the blood. Homocysteine is produced when red meat and dairy products are broken down in the body and high levels of homocysteine give an increased risk of heart attacks and strokes.

**Vitamin C acts as a diuretic, which helps, remove sodium and water from the body which in turn helps relax blood vessel walls and decrease blood pressure. Vitamin C also helps the body develop resistance to infectious agents.

* **Vitamin D** acts similar to ACE inhibitors in reducing high blood pressure. Studies have shown that people with low levels of vitamin D are more likely to have high blood pressure.

So how do you find out what is in the foods you buy? One way is to learn how to read the labels on the packaged foods you buy. The Recommended Dietary Allowance (RDA) label contains information you need to make an informed choice. You want to purchase items with lower percentage numbers on fats, cholesterol, sodium, and added sugars. You want to purchase items with higher percentage numbers on fiber, vitamins, and minerals. The FDA is updating the requirements for these labels in 2016. An explanation of the label and the new change requirements can be found at:

http://www.fda.gov/Food/GuidanceRegulation/GuidanceDocument sRegulatoryInformation/LabelingNutrition/ucm385663.htm

~~~~~~~~~~

Recommended Items For Control or Reduction of High Blood Pressure

Again - if you want to maintain healthy blood pressure levels, what foods should you eat that have these minerals, vitamins, and nutrients? This "What To Eat" section is broken down into the categories of Vegetables, Fruits, Beans, Nuts, Fish, Dairy, Herbs and Spices, Supplements, and Other. In the categories, I have concentrated on listing foods that are high in one or more these minerals, vitamins and/or nutrients. Each food listed has some brief information about it, how much of the Recommended Dietary Allowance for the needed nutrients it contains, and/or suggested ideas on ways to increase the food in your diet. In each category, if the item in a category had less than 1% of the daily RDA for one of the important nutrients, then that nutrient was not in the RDA list for that item. Even though other nutrients may be obtained in an item, only the ones identified as being important to blood pressure control are in the RDA list.

~~~~~~~~~~

Vegetables

The American Heart Association recommends nine servings (about 4.5 cups) of fruits and vegetables be eaten every day. Vegetables contain vitamins and fiber, and many are rich in potassium, calcium, and/or magnesium that work to keep your body and blood pressure in good condition. Some vegetables, particularly green leafy vegetables, are a good source for increasing nitric oxide levels in blood. Nitric oxide is a vasodilator that causes the muscles in the blood vessel walls to relax which in turn causes the vessels to dilate (widen) and allows the blood to flow with less pressure.

Canned and frozen vegetables can be comparable to fresh in nutritional values as long as they do not contain added sugars and fats, artificial preservatives, or excessive amounts of added sodium.

* Asparagus - Asparagus has been considered a delicacy since ancient times. It is a perennial plant with succulent tall herbaceous stems and flowery foliage. It is high in anti-inflammatory and antioxidant nutrients. Asparagus is also known as a natural diuretic.

One cup of asparagus provides the following daily Recommended Dietary Allowance (RDA) for Vitamin C 12%, Potassium 7%, Vitamin B-6 5%, Magnesium 4%, and Calcium 3%.

Ways to increase asparagus in your diet...

Eat asparagus as a side dish - blanch, steam, simmer, bake, roast, grill, or sauté; in vegetable stir fry; in chicken stir fry, in shrimp stir fry; cream of asparagus soup; roasted with cherry tomatoes; sautéed with mushrooms; roasted with new potatoes; asparagus and onion casserole; in a salad with strawberries and baby spinach, in a salad with goat cheese and quinoa; in a salad with tomato and avocado;...

* Beetroot - Beetroot is the root portion of the beet plant. Beetroot should not be confused with the sugar beet. The rootstock of a beet is normally red or gold in color unlike the sugar beet that is white in color. You may want to wear rubber/vinyl gloves when preparing beets because their color can leave a stubborn stain on your hands. Beetroot is rich in antioxidants and is also a good source for increasing nitric oxide levels in the blood. If you purchase fresh beets with the leaves still attached, do not discard the leaves as they are also packed with vitamins and minerals. Use them in salads or prepare them the same as you would with other green leafy vegetables. Note that the dark color of the beetroot juice may cause color changes to your urine or stool. This is normal and can occur if the beets are consumed either raw or cooked.

One cup of beetroot provides the following daily RDA for Potassium 12%, Vitamin C 11%, Magnesium 7%, Vitamin B-6 5%, Sodium 4%, and Calcium 2%.

Ways to increase beetroot in your diet...

Eat beets as a side dish raw, roasted, steamed, or boiled; in a mixed green salad with radish, onions, and celery; beet soup made with beet, onion, and garlic; beetroot and carrot soup; grated raw in salads; beetroot and cabbage slaw; roasted beetroot and quinoa salad; beetroot and asparagus salad; beetroot and potato puree; beetroot and butternut squash stew;...

Drink: Because of the potency of beetroot juice, the potential side effects (one of which is an increased risk for developing kidney or gallstones), and the susceptibility of having harmful bacteria in the juice, I do not recommend drinking of juiced beetroot;....

* **Bok Choy** - Bok Choy (also known as Chinese white cabbage) is a cruciferous vegetable cultivated for thousands of years. It is loaded with blood pressure reducing minerals. The top of bok choy resembles Romaine lettuce and the bottom resembles large celery, but bok choy is a cruciferous vegetable more closely related to cabbage. Potassium, calcium, and magnesium are all present in bok choy. Bok choy is known for its mild flavor and can be eaten raw like celery.

One cup of bok choy provides the following daily RDA for Vitamin C 52%, Calcium 7%, Potassium 5%, Vitamin B-6 5%, Magnesium 3%, and Sodium 1%.

Ways to increase bok choy in your diet...

Eat bok choy raw, steamed, boiled, or stir fried; use bok choy in place of red or green cabbage in recipes; raw in a salad with green onions, almonds, and sesame seeds; stir fried with garlic; bok choy slaw with carrots and scallions; bok choy soup with shrimp and mushrooms; bok choy chicken soup; stir fry chicken and bok choy; stir fry with carrots, broccoli and cauliflower; steamed pumpkin and bok choy and ginger; steamed bok choy and broccoli;...

* **Broccoli** - Broccoli is in the cabbage family and like bok choy is a cruciferous vegetable. It is one of the most popular vegetables in the USA. Broccoli is loaded with Vitamin C. Broccoli is also rich in other vitamins, minerals, and antioxidants. If you like the taste of broccoli, it is more nutritious if eaten raw.

One cup of broccoli provides the following daily RDA for Vitamin C 135%, Vitamin B-6 10%, Potassium 8%, Calcium 4%, Magnesium 4%, and Sodium 1%.

Ways to increase broccoli in your diet...

Eat broccoli raw, steamed, roasted, baked, or stir fried; raw in salads; broccoli cole slaw; broccoli, raisins, red onion, and sunflower seed salad; sautéed broccoli, green bean, and corn; steamed broccoli with cashews; stir fried sesame broccoli; stir fried broccoli and kale; broccoli with mandarin orange; stir fried broccoli, snow peas, red onion, and bell pepper; roasted broccoli salad; baked broccoli, pumpkin, beet, onion, sweet potato, and red potato;...

* **Brussel sprouts** - Brussel sprouts look like miniature cabbages. French settlers brought it to the United States in the early 1800's. It is a cruciferous vegetable with a nutty, earthy taste and is rich in vitamins, minerals, and antioxidants. Green sprouts with a white base are fresher than those with a base that is slightly yellow or brown.

One cup of brussel sprouts provides the following daily RDA for Vitamin C 124%, Vitamin B-6 10%, Potassium 9%, Magnesium 5%, and Calcium 3%

Ways to increase brussel sprouts in your diet...

Eat brussel sprouts raw, steamed, roasted, boiled, stir fried, or grilled; chopped brussel sprout, kale, and dried fruit salad; roasted brussel sprouts and grapes; roasted brussel sprouts with pecans; stir fried brussel sprouts, apricots and almonds; garlic roasted salmon and brussel sprouts; roasted brussel sprouts and shallots; wild rice pilaf with sweet potatoes and brussel sprouts; apple and pistachio brussel sprout salad;...

* **Cabbage** - Cabbage originated in Asia and was domesticated in Europe around 1000 BC. There are many different varieties of cabbage, but for this category, we are talking about the most commonly identified cabbages which are the densely leaved green and red/purple cabbages. Cabbage is loaded with vitamins in addition to having the important minerals needed for high blood pressure control.

One cup of chopped cabbage provides the following daily RDA for Vitamin C 54%, Vitamin B-6 5%, Potassium 4%, Calcium 3%, and Magnesium 2%.

Ways to increase cabbage in your diet...

Eat cabbage raw, steamed, roasted, boiled, stir fried, or grilled; cabbage slaw; grilled cabbage wedges, fish tacos with cabbage slaw; apple cabbage salad or slaw; cabbage, carrots, onions, tomatoes, peppers, and celery soup; stewed cabbage with tomato, onion, celery, and garlic; boiled sweet and sour red cabbage and apples; stir fried cabbage, tofu and red pepper; turnip and cabbage slaw; sautéed shredded cabbage and squash; broccoli, cabbage and kohlrabi coleslaw; potato and cabbage soup; oven baked red cabbage chips; cabbage salsa; red cabbage and brussel sprouts pizza;...

* **Carrots** - Carrots are root vegetables that come in a variety of colors but the orange colored carrot is the most familiar. Carrots come in many lengths, 2 inches to as long as 3 feet. Carrots are rich in beta-carotene, which once ingested is converted into vitamin A. Carrots have not only beta-carotene but also alpha-carotene and studies show that diets high in carotenoids are associated with lower risks for heart disease. According to a study at Harvard University, people who ate five or more carrots a week

are less likely to suffer a stroke than those who eat only one carrot a month or less.

One cup of chopped carrots provides the following daily RDA for Vitamin C 12%, Potassium 11%, Vitamin B-6 10%, Calcium 4%, Magnesium 3%, and Sodium 3%.

Ways to increase carrots in your diet...

Eat carrots raw, steamed, roasted, boiled, stir fried, glazed, or grilled; cooked with green peas, carrot and raisin salad; chopped, sliced, or grated in a green or fruit salad; cooked with bok choy and green beans; carrot and cabbage slaw; roasted with turmeric and cumin; mashed carrots and potato; mashed carrots and cauliflower; roasted carrots, potatoes, and brussel sprouts; carrot, onion, and celery puree; stir fry with garlic and ginger; stir fry with mushrooms and green onion; stir fry with a combination of other vegetables like broccoli, corn, green beans, snow peas, celery, bell peppers, onions, etc; carrot and herbs soup; boiled carrots and celery;...

* **Celery** -Celery is a vegetable that has been cultivated globally for centuries and is another vegetable that is high in anti-inflammatory and antioxidant nutrients. Celery is used in many salads and cooked dishes but is probably best known as a low calorie but filling snack. Celery stored at room temperature will quickly become limp. To preserve it longer, celery should be refrigerated. Celery should be wrapped tightly in aluminum foil and stored in the refrigerator. Do not store it in an airtight plastic storage bag or container. This is because celery releases a ripening hormone (ethylene). Aluminum foil wrap allows the ethylene to escape but an airtight container will cause the celery to go limp more quickly than being stored open at room temperature. Wrapping in aluminum foil is the method I use and have found that it works great.

One cup of chopped celery provides the following daily RDA for Potassium 7%, Vitamin B-6 5%, Vitamin C 5%, Calcium 4%, Sodium 3%, and Magnesium 2%.

Ways to increase celery in your diet...

Eat celery raw, steamed, roasted, boiled, stir fried, or grilled; celery, cabbage, and onion slaw; celery and apple slaw; chop, slice, or grate in a green or fruit salad; celery and beet salad; stir fry with a combination of other vegetables like broccoli, corn, green beans, carrots, snow peas, bell peppers, onions, etc.; stir fry with other vegetables and cashews, almonds, sunflower seeds, or pumpkin seeds; celery, potato, and onion soup; celery and apple soup; boiled celery and carrots; celery and almond butter;...

* **Cauliflower** - Cauliflower like broccoli is also cruciferous vegetable. It is more popular China and India than broccoli is in the United States. While the most common color for cauliflower is white, it also comes in orange, purple, and green. The green leaves of the cauliflower are edible but most often they are discarded. This is a waste since the leaves and stem of the cauliflower also contain vital nutrients. Cauliflower can also serve as a reasonable lower starch substitute for potatoes or rice in some dishes.

One cup of chopped cauliflower provides the following daily RDA for Vitamin C 85%, Vitamin B-6 10%, Potassium 9%, Magnesium 4%, Calcium 2%, and Sodium 1%.

Ways to increase cauliflower in your diet...

Eat cauliflower raw, steamed, roasted, boiled, stir fried, or grilled; cauliflower and tomato salad; cauliflower and broccoli salad; cauliflower, broccoli, carrot, strawberries, and almonds salad; cauliflower roasted with pumpkin seeds; roasted with brussel sprouts, apples, onion then added walnuts and raisins; boiled with green peas; stir fried with a combination of other vegetables like broccoli, corn, green beans, carrots, snow peas, celery, bell peppers, onions, etc; chopped, sliced, or grated in a green salad; cauliflower and chives soup; mashed cauliflower; cauliflower and carrot soup; roasted with potatoes, carrots, beets, and shallot;...

* **Cucumber** - Cucumber belongs to the same family as melons and squash. Although generally referred to as a vegetable, technically since the cucumber grows from the flower of the plant, it is a fruit. Cucumbers contain anti-inflammatory compounds as

well as being filled with Vitamin C, a powerful antioxidant, and other nutrients essential to natural blood pressure control. Cucumber is also a natural diuretic.

One cucumber (a little over 8" long) provides the following daily RDA for Vitamin C 14%, Potassium 12%, Magnesium 9%, Vitamin B-6 5%, and Calcium 4%.

Ways to increase cucumber in your diet...

Most cucumber recipes call for raw cucumbers but cucumbers can be eaten raw, steamed, roasted, or stir fried; chop or slice cucumbers in a green or fruit salad; cucumber and tomato sandwich; cucumber, celery, and tuna salad; cucumber, zucchini, onion and garlic soup; steamed cucumber with tomato; roasted cucumber with onions; stir fry with ginger; drink water infused with cucumber; pickled cumbers are common but unfortunately pickled cucumbers contain a large amount of sodium and should not be eaten by those with high blood pressure;...

* **Eggplant** - The edible part of the eggplant is a fruit even though most people would call them a vegetable. Because of the eggplant belongs to the nightshade family of plants, its flowers and leaves can be poisonous if consumed in large enough quantities. The best-known and most popular variety of eggplant has an elongated pear shape and a deep purple skin. Eggplants are also available in other shapes and sizes as well as in a variety of colors. In some dishes, eggplants can be used as a meat substitute. Since the raw fruit can sometimes have a bitter taste, the most common way to eat eggplant is cooked.

One eggplant (1+lbs) with peel provides the following daily RDA for Potassium 35%, Vitamin B-6 25%, Vitamin C 20%, Magnesium 19%, and Calcium 4%.

Ways to increase eggplant in your diet...

Eat eggplant baked, boiled, roasted, stir fried, or steamed; baked eggplant and tomato; roasted eggplant, onions, and sweet peppers; stir-fry eggplant with vegetables; boiled chopped eggplant seasoned with herbs and spices; oven baked eggplant fries; oven baked eggplant chips; eggplant, white bean, and onion soup;

grilled eggplant topped with tomato and onion salsa; eggplant, zucchini, and tomato casserole; steamed eggplant, onions, and sweet peppers;...

* **Fennel** - Fennel is a flowering plant species in the carrot family. Fennel has a white or pale green bulb with closely group stalks growing upward from the bulb. The stalks have feathery green leaves and flowers that produce fennel seeds. The bulb, stalk, leaves, and seeds are all edible. Fennel has a mild but distinctive licorice flavor and can be used in much the same way as celery.

One cup of sliced fennel provides the following daily RDA for Vitamin C 17%, Potassium 10%, Calcium 4%, and Magnesium 3%.

Ways to increase fennel in your diet...

Eat fennel raw, steamed, roasted, boiled, stir fried, or grilled; fennel soup; fennel in a salad with watercress, radicchio and pecan; in a salad with grapefruit, avocado, onion, and romaine lettuce; fennel and cucumber salsa; fennel, arugula, black olives, and sliced orange salad; roasted fennel, beets, and apples; fennel and tomato soup; stir fried with a combination of other vegetables like broccoli, corn, green beans, carrots, snow peas, celery, bell peppers, onions, etc; roasted fennel with tomatoes, olives, and potatoes; fennel, zucchini, and onion soup;...

* **Garlic** - Garlic is a vegetable bulb that belongs to the lily family and is a close relative to leeks, chives, and onions. Instead of being the main ingredient in a recipe, it is generally used as a flavoring ingredient in recipes rather than as the main ingredient itself. I personally have found that I like the texture of minced or chopped garlic in recipes much more than using garlic powder. Garlic contains a substance called allicin. Allicin has antibacterial, antioxidant, lipid lowering and anti-hypertensive properties.

Fresh garlic: Three (3) cloves of garlic (an average garlic bulb has about 10 cloves) provide the following daily RDA for Vitamin B-6 5%, Vitamin C 4%, Calcium 1%, and Potassium 1%.

Garlic powder: One (1) teaspoon of provides Vitamin B-6 5%, and Potassium 1%. It also contains Vitamin C and Calcium but provides less than 1% of each of these.

Ways to increase fresh garlic in your diet...

Even though dry ground garlic powder is commonly used as a flavoring ingredient, chopped or minced garlic cloves can also be used in the following: garlic, onion, and tomato salsa; minced garlic in mashed potatoes; chopped or minced garlic in stir fry dishes; roasted garlic spread on toasted whole grain bread; sautéed kale and chopped garlic; minced garlic, green peas and onions; minced garlic in mashed cauliflower; garlic and basil pesto; minced garlic, cucumber, avocado, cilantro and onion salad; stir fried garlic, tofu, and eggplant; sautéed garlic, onions, and kale; sautéed garlic as a side dish; garlic soup;...

* Leafy Greens - Kale, turnip greens, and spinach are well known examples of leafy greens. Leafy greens are a major dietary source for heart healthy vitamins and minerals. Kale has been grown and eaten for thousands of years but began to lose its popularity to cabbage during the Middle Ages. Turnips and turnip greens were a well-established food by Roman times but spinach came from central or southwestern Asia and was not known in Europe until after about 800 AD.

Kale - One cup of chopped kale provides the following daily RDA for Vitamin C 134%, Calcium 10%, Vitamin B-6 10%, Potassium 9%, Magnesium 7%, and Sodium 1%.

Turnip Greens - One cup of chopped turnip greens provides the following daily RDA for Vitamin C 65%, Calcium 19%, Vitamin B-6 15%, Magnesium 8%, Potassium 8%, and Sodium 1%.

Spinach - One cup of spinach provides the following daily RDA for Vitamin C 14%, Magnesium 6%, Vitamin B-6 5%, Potassium 4%, Calcium 3%, and Sodium 1%.

Romaine lettuce, Swiss chard, mustard greens, collard greens, watercress, arugula, and other leafy greens are also high in vitamins and minerals. Unlike many of the other vegetables in this list, even though leafy greens can be eaten raw, you get the more benefits related to blood pressure when the greens are cooked.

Ways to increase leafy greens in your diet...

Eat leafy greens raw, steamed, roasted, boiled, stir fried, or grilled; baked or microwaved kale chips; kale with sunflower seeds, tomatoes, and cranberries salad; roasted kale and beet salad; kale, vegetable, and bean soup; steamed kale with minced garlic; kale, bean, and potato soup; stir fried kale, onion, and garlic; classic boiled turnip greens; turnip greens soup; sautéed turnip greens, pine nuts, and raisins; mashed turnips and potatoes with steamed turnip greens; spinach and mushroom stir fry; roasted spinach and sweet potatoes; baked spinach chips; spinach, cranberry, and almond salad;...

* **Onion** - Even though there is no definitive proof, it is believed that our earliest ancestors started eating wild onions long before farming was invented. Though Yellow onions comprise 75% of the world's production of onions, there are over 30 varieties of onions including: Leeks, Pearl Onions, Red Onions, Scallion, Shallots, Spring Onions, Vidalias, Walla Walla; White Onions, and others. Onions are filled with quercetin that is a powerful antioxidant flavonol effective in reducing blood pressure. Either raw or cooked onions contain good natural sources of nutrients that reduce high blood pressure, but some studies show that raw onions are more effective than cooked ones.

One cup of chopped raw onion provides the following daily RDA for Vitamin C 19%, Vitamin B-6 10%, Potassium 6%, Magnesium 4%, and Calcium 3%.

Ways to increase onions in your diet...

Eat onions raw, steamed, roasted, boiled, stir fried, or grilled; chopped or sliced onions in a green or fruit salad; baked sweet onion; grilled onions and potatoes; English peas and pearl onions; onion roasted sweet potatoes; onion soup; stir fry with a combination of other vegetables like broccoli, corn, green beans, carrots, snow peas, bell peppers, celery, etc.; onion, mushroom, garlic gravy; onions as a topping on baked potatoes; almond glazed onions; grilled onion blossom; glazed pearl onions with raisins and almonds; roasted red onion, beet, and purple carrot; roasted onion and cucumber; onion, corn, and bell pepper pudding; oven baked onion rings;...

* **Potatoes** - There are over 100 varieties within the seven categories of potatoes sold in the US. These categories are blue/purple, fingerling, petite, red, russet, white, and yellow potatoes. The russet potato (or Idaho potato) is the type most readily identified as the classic potato. Potatoes are the number one vegetable crop in the world. The potato's starchy tuber is very high in potassium and magnesium, and is rich source for other vitamins and minerals. Because of the potential for gastric problems, it is recommended that potatoes not be eaten raw and uncooked. French fries and potato chips cooked in boiling oil are also not recommended for those trying to maintain and control their blood pressure levels.

One large russet potato (3" - 4" dia) provides the following daily RDA for Vitamin B-6 65%, Potassium 43%, Vitamin C 35%, Magnesium 21%, and Calcium 4%.

Ways to increase potato in your diet...

Eat white potatoes baked, boiled, roasted, or steamed; classic whole baked potato (without salty toppings); mashed potatoes with scallions; garlic roasted potatoes; potato soup (hot or cold); oven baked, microwaved, or dehydrated potato chips without oil; potatoes steamed with garlic, green onion, and parsley; baked cubed potatoes and vegetables like squash, zucchini, bell pepper; onions, and/or carrots; oven baked French "fries" seasoned with herbs and spices;...

* **Potatoes – Sweet** - A sweet potato is a large, sweet tasting, starchy a root vegetable. It is thought that sweet potatoes originated in either Central or South America more than 5000 years ago. The most common and best-known sweet potatoes have a reddish pink or orange colored flesh and in some parts of the United States are often referred to as a yam.

One cup of cubed sweet potato provides the following daily RDA for Vitamin B-6 15%, Potassium 12%, Magnesium 8%, Vitamin C 5%, Calcium 4%, and Sodium 3%.

Ways to increase sweet potatoes in your diet...

Sweet potatoes can be eaten raw, baked, boiled, roasted, stir fried, or steamed; raw sweet potato and kale salad; raw grated sweet potato, celery, and apple salad; mashed sweet potato; roasted sweet potato and carrots; roasted sweet potato and cauliflower salad; sweet potato pie; stir fried sweet potato, broccoli, and peppers; oven baked, microwaved, or dehydrated sweet potato chips without using oil; sweet potato soup;...

* **Pumpkin** - The well-known pumpkin is actually part of the winter squash family. Pumpkins are believed to have originated in the ancient Americas and American Indians introduced pumpkins to the Pilgrims. The pumpkin is more than just a Halloween decoration. It is low in calories but high in healthy antioxidants, vitamins, and minerals. Pureed or canned pumpkin can be used as a healthier substitute for eggs and oil in many baked goods recipes. If you buy canned pumpkin just make sure it is not pumpkin pie filling and that it does not have added sugars, salt, and/or other preservatives.

One cup of cubed pumpkin provides the following daily RDA for Vitamin C 17%, Potassium 11%, Vitamin B-6 5%, Magnesium 3%, and Calcium 2%.

Ways to increase pumpkin in your diet..

Pumpkins can be eaten raw, baked, boiled, roasted, stir fried, or steamed; pumpkin and cauliflower casserole; stir fried pumpkin, brussel sprouts, and apples; roasted pumpkin in green salad with peaches and almonds; roasted pumpkin soup with mushrooms and onions; pumpkin and carrot soup; pureed pumpkin in oatmeal; mashed pumpkin and potatoes; dried or roasted pumpkin seeds;...

* **Squash** - Summer squash (yellow squash and zucchini being the most common) and Winter squash (acorn, butternut squash, and

pumpkin being the most common) are usually available in markets year round. They were given the summer and winter designations in a time when the seasons dictated what was available on the farm and in local markets.

Summer squash - One cup of sliced summer squash provides the following daily RDA for Vitamin C 32%, Vitamin B-6 10%, Potassium 8%, Magnesium 4%, and Calcium 1%.

Winter squash - One cup of cubed winter squash provides the following daily RDA for Vitamin C 23%, Potassium 11%, Vitamin B-6 10%, Magnesium 4%, and Calcium 3%.

Ways to increase squash in your diet...

Squash can be eaten raw, baked, boiled, roasted, stir fried, or steamed; raw sliced or grated summer squash in a green salad; raw summer squash and tomato salad; oven roasted summer squash with onion, garlic, and bell pepper; oven roasted zucchini, yellow squash, potato, onion, and tomato casserole; roasted winter squash, carrots, turnips, and sweet potatoes; steamed yellow squash and sweet onion; steamed summer squash and broccoli; grilled squash, eggplant, zucchini, and onion; roasted butternut squash soup;...

* **Tomatoes** - Tomatoes, like eggplants, are fruits that are usually thought of as a being a vegetable. Even though the tomato plant is a member of the deadly nightshade family, the tomato fruit is one of the world's healthiest foods filled with vitamins, minerals, and antioxidants. Tomatoes are America's favorite home garden plant and they come in many sizes, shapes, colors, and flavors. Some are tart and others are very sweet. Some are juicier and some have less juice and a thicker flesh. Tomatoes should not be stored in the refrigerator because that spoils the flavor and taste. Tomatoes can be frozen for 8 to 12 months but they will be mushy when thawed and frozen tomatoes are best if used in cooked recipes. If you grow them yourself or have a nearby farmers market, water bath canning of tomatoes is also an easy way to preserve them for future use.

One cup of chopped or sliced red tomato provides the following daily RDA for Vitamin C 41%, Potassium 12%, Magnesium 5%, Vitamin B-6 5%, and Calcium 1%.

Ways to increase tomato in your diet...

Eat: raw sliced tomatoes; raw cherry tomatoes as a snack; tomatoes in green salads or fruit salads; as an ingredient in many salsa recipes; tomato and vegetable stir-fry; roasted cherry tomatoes; grilled green or ripe tomatoes; roasted tomato sauce; tomato soup; boiled tomatoes and vegetables; tomatoes and vegetable casserole; tomatoes and vegetable soup; tomato sauce; homemade tomato ketchup (made with honey instead of sugar); oven dried or dehydrated tomatoes;...

Drink: tomato juice;...

~~~~~~~~~~

Fruits

In addition to being colorful and full of flavors, fruits contain minerals, vitamins, and anti-oxidants needed for natural maintenance and control of blood pressure. Fruits are noted as being an excellent source for Vitamin C. Vitamin C acts as a diuretic that helps remove sodium and water from the body thus helping relax blood vessel walls and decreasing blood pressure. Most fruits are edible in their raw form and consuming raw fruit usually gives you their maximum fruit nutrition. Most fruits can also be dried or cooked. In many cases, dried fruit provides a higher concentration per ounce of the nutrients most needed to maintain health blood pressure. Just be sure if you eat dried fruits that they are prepared without added sweeteners or sulphites. I had already purchased and have used a dehydrator and have found it easy to make my own dried fruits and I know that they do not have these problematic additives. Many plants commonly considered as vegetables are technically fruits. Tomatoes, eggplant, and squash (all listed in the above vegetable section) are examples of fruits commonly referred to as vegetables.

* **Apples** - Everyone knows the old saying "an apple a day keeps the doctor away". Apples contain flavonoids that are important

antioxidants that help protect blood vessels from damage and in maintaining healthy blood pressure. Apples are filled with quercetin that is a powerful antioxidant flavonol that is effective in reducing blood pressure. Apples are also a good source of Vitamin C and Potassium.

One medium size apple (3" dia) provides the following daily RDA for Vitamin C 14%, Potassium 5%, Vitamin B-6 5%, Magnesium 2%, and Calcium 1%.

Ways to increase apples in your diet...

Eat: fresh apples with or without skin; slices of apple added to hot oatmeal or cereal; unsweetened applesauce; apple butter (made without sugar); dried apple chips; baked apples; apples in a fruit salad; apples in a green salad; apple, raisin, and carrot salad; apple and vegetable stir-fry; roasted apple, carrots, onion, cauliflower, and sweet potato; apple, onion, and beet soup; apple, cabbage, and radish slaw;...

Drink: unsweetened apple juice; unsweetened apple cider;...

* **Apricots** - Apricots are closely related to peaches and plums, and apricots have as much potassium as bananas. In addition to needed minerals, they are also a good source of heart healthy antioxidants such as beta-carotene (Vitamin A) and Vitamin C. One cup of sliced apricots provides the following daily RDA for Vitamin C 27%, Potassium 12%, Vitamin B-6 5%, Magnesium 4%, and Calcium 2%.

Ways to increase apricots in your diet...

Eat: fresh apricots whole or sliced; sliced apricots in hot or cold cereal; fresh apricots in a fruit salad; fresh apricots in a green salad; apricots in yogurt; cooked apricot soup sweetened with honey (chill before serving); apricot, pineapple, and vegetable stir-fry; honey roasted apricots; dried apricots; dried apricot bits in granola mixes;...

Drink: apricot juice (without added sugars, preservatives, and/or other additives);...

* **Avocado** - The avocado is sometimes called an "alligator pear" because of its shape and green, bumpy skin. Avocados also contain a lot more potassium than bananas. Avocado is a high fat food but it is a monounsaturated fat not the unhealthy trans fat and refined polyunsaturated fat found in most processed foods. Some studies show that the type of fat found in the avocado increases vitamin and antioxidant absorption from other foods eaten with avocado. Always remove the large pit as preparation for eating avocado.

One cup of sliced avocado provides the following daily RDA for Vitamin C 24%, Potassium 20%, Vitamin B-6 20%, Magnesium 10%, and Calcium 1%.

Ways to increase avocados in your diet...

Eat: avocados are best used raw, but they can be cooked; raw sliced avocado topped with olive oil, black pepper, and lemon juice; guacamole (avocado dip); avocado soup; fresh avocado in a fruit salad; fresh avocado in a green salad; avocado, cucumber, and peach salad; avocado and black bean salsa; avocado, cucumber, and onion soup (chill before serving); grilled avocado; oven baked avocado fries; substitute mashed avocado for mayonnaise or sour cream; avocado and vegetable stir-fry;...

* **Banana** - Bananas are one of the first fruits that come to mind when thinking about blood pressure control. That is because of the high potassium content found in bananas. Bananas may be the most widely consumed fruit in the world. Once a banana is ripe, it can be stored for several days in the refrigerator. The skin of ripe bananas quickly blackens in the refrigerator but the fruit inside remains unaffected. Note that once an un-ripened banana is refrigerated it will not ripen further even when removed from the refrigerator. Peeled or pureed bananas can be stored in a freezer bag in the freezer for about 2 months. Adding lemon juice before freezing will prevent discoloration. Another note is that apples will accelerate the ripening process of bananas, so do not put them on the counter together.

One medium banana (7"-8" Long) provides the following daily RDA for Vitamin B-6 20%, Vitamin C 17%, Potassium 12%, and Magnesium 8%.

Ways to increase bananas in your diet...

Eat: the number 1 method is peel a raw, ripe banana and eat it; sliced bananas in hot or cold cereal; banana and almond butter sandwich on whole grain bread; oven baked or dehydrated banana chips; frozen sliced bananas and almond butter snack; banana and mango salsa; frozen banana popsicle; banana spread made with honey; sugar-less banana bread made with whole wheat flour; bananas, oats, walnuts, raisins, and sunflower seed snack bars;...

* Berries (Blackberry, Blueberry, Strawberry) - Wild berries have been a food source for humans since prehistoric days. Different varieties of berries have been domesticated and cultivated for thousands of years. The three varieties listed here are filled with anti-oxidants, vitamins and/or minerals needed for healthy blood pressure control. Other varieties of berries also have many of these in varying amounts. Berries come in many colors and it is thought that the color attracts birds and animals that consume the berries and thus spread the seed. The chemicals that give berries their colors also give berries a high anti-oxidant content.

Blackberries - One cup of blackberries provides the following daily RDA for Vitamin C 50%, Magnesium 7%, Potassium 6%, and Calcium 4%.

Blueberry - One cup of blueberries provides the following daily RDA for Vitamin C 24%, Vitamin B-6 5%, Potassium 3%, and Magnesium 2%.

Strawberries - One cup of strawberries provides the following daily RDA for Vitamin C 162%, Potassium 7%, Magnesium 5%, Vitamin B-6 5%, and Calcium 2%.

Ways to increase berries in your diet...

Eat: berries raw as a snack; berries in hot or cold cereal; berries in a fruit salad, berries in a green salad; dried or dehydrated berries;

stir-fried berries and vegetables; dried berries and toasted barley granola; berry and boiled/steamed asparagus; honey sweetened berry sauce; honey sweetened berry preserves; as a topping on nonfat yogurt;...

* Figs - Figs were cultivated in ancient Egypt. Fresh figs have a short shelf life and even if refrigerated will only stay fresh for a few days. The process of drying can preserve figs longer. As you can see by the listing below, drying figs greatly increases the mineral concentration per cup of figs. Dried figs have a much longer shelf life (up to several months) if kept in a cool, dark place or in the refrigerator. Dried figs can be used as is in many recipes or re-hydrated to make them juicier.

Fresh figs - two/thirds of a cup of fresh figs provides the following daily RDA for Potassium 6%, Vitamin B-6 5%, Magnesium 4%, Calcium 3%, and Vitamin C 3%.

Dried figs - two/thirds of a cup of dried figs provides the following daily RDA for Potassium 19%, Magnesium 17%, Calcium 16%, Vitamin B-6 5%, and Vitamin C 2%.

Ways to increase figs in your diet...

Figs can be eaten fresh, cooked, or dried; fresh figs with yogurt, honey, and nuts; fig, watermelon, and onion salad; grilled fig in green salads or fruit salads; roasted fig, beet, and walnut salad; fig, kale, avocado, and cashew salad; roasted figs and brussel sprouts; figs as a topping in oatmeal; roasted figs and potatoes; figs and walnuts with roasted sweet potatoes; fig stuffed baked apples;...

* Kiwifruit - A cup of sliced kiwifruit (also known as Chinese gooseberry) has much more Vitamin C, potassium, and magnesium than a cup of orange sections. The peel of the kiwifruit is a fuzzy brownish/green and the shape and size of the fruit resembles a chicken egg. The inside flesh of the fruit is bright green with tiny black seed around the core. Kiwifruit is a good source of heart healthy minerals, antioxidants, and omega-3 fatty acids.

One cup of sliced kiwi provides the following daily RDA for Vitamin C 278%, Potassium 16%, Magnesium 7%, Calcium 6%, and Vitamin B-6 5%.

Ways to increase kiwifruit in your diet...

Kiwifruit is usually peeled and consumed raw; kiwifruit peeled and sliced; kiwifruit, grapefruit, and blueberry salad; kiwifruit and shredded cabbage salad; kiwifruit in green salads or fruit salads;...

* Mango - Known as the "king of fruits" the mango is believed to have originated in India. The mango fruit's juicy orange-yellow flesh is rich in vitamins, minerals, and antioxidants. Mangoes are one of the most commonly eaten fruits in the tropical countries of the world. Once completely ripe, mangoes, can be stored in a refrigerator for up to 5 days and ripe sliced or cubed mangoes can be stored in the freezer in airtight containers for 6 to 10 months.

One average size peeled and de-stoned mango provides the following daily RDA for Vitamin C 203%, Vitamin B-6 20%, Potassium 16%, Magnesium 8%, and Calcium 3%.

Ways to increase mango in your diet...

Like many other fruits, a mango is usually peeled and consumed raw but can also be cooked or dried; mangoes in green salads or fruit salads; mango, avocado, tomato, and onion salsa; stir-fry mangoes, bell peppers, mushrooms, and broccoli; baked mango and honey; cooked mango and honey pudding; grilled mangoes; fresh mango slices as a topping in oatmeal; oven dried mango slices or bits;...

* Melon - Cantaloupe and Honeydew - There are many varieties of melons with edible sweet flesh inside the melon rind. For this segment, we will talk about two of the most readily available melons - the cantaloupe and the honeydew melon. The watermelon will be covered in a separate section. Some researchers think the melon originated in Africa, others think it was in southern Asia. In either case, melons began to appear in Europe towards the end of the Roman Empire. Melons are over 90% water but they are also nutrient filled with vitamins and minerals.

Cantaloupe - One cup of cubed cantaloupe provides the following daily RDA for Vitamin C 97%, Potassium 12%, Vitamin B-6 5%, Magnesium 4%, Calcium 1%, and Sodium 1%.

Honeydew melon - One cup of cubed honeydew melon provides the following daily RDA for Vitamin C 51%, Potassium 11%, Vitamin B-6 5%, Magnesium 4%, Calcium 1%, and Sodium 1%.

Ways to increase cantaloupe and honeydew melon in your diet...

Melons are generally eaten raw but can also be an ingredient in cooked recipes; melons (rind and seeds removed) sliced, cubed, or balled; melons in green salads or fruit salads; cantaloupe, cucumber, tomato, and onion salsa; raw pureed cantaloupe or honeydew melon, cucumber, and onion soup (gazpacho, serve chilled); roasted cantaloupe; raw pureed honeydew melon and blueberry soup (serve chilled); grilled cantaloupe and honey;...

* **Oranges** - The orange is probably the world's most popular citrus fruit. With the advances in processing and transportation, widespread consumption of oranges became possible in America during the 20th century. Before that in the USA, because of the expense and lack of availability, oranges were usually eaten on special holidays such as Christmas. A recent World Health Organization report said that a diet that includes citrus fruits offers protection against cardiovascular disease. The report attributes the citrus fruit's high levels of potassium as well as vitamin C, carotenoids, and flavonoids. All of these have been identified as having protective cardiovascular effects.

One cup of orange sections provides the following daily RDA for Vitamin C 159%, Potassium 9%, Calcium 7%, Vitamin B-6 5%, and Magnesium 4%.

Ways to increase oranges in your diet...

Eat: the most common method to eat oranges is just to peel and eat (raw gives the most health benefits); orange segments in green salads or fruit salads; orange juice used as a flavoring agent in many different recipes; roasted beets with orange segments; oranges roasted with honey and cinnamon; roasted orange and asparagus; roasted orange, potatoes, carrots and turnip; oven dried or dehydrated orange wheels;...

Drink: Fresh squeezed orange juice; bottled, cartoned, or frozen orange juice (just make sure there are no added sugars, preservatives, and/or other additives)...

* **Pomegranate** - One of the earliest cultivated fruits was the pomegranate. The antioxidants in pomegranates along with high amounts of potassium and magnesium give pomegranates their blood pressure reducing properties. The edible parts of a pomegranate are the seeds and the white pithy part surrounding the seeds. The outer skin is tough and is not eaten. Pomegranates have a sweet-tart flavor that makes them a favorite ingredient in many recipes.

One pomegranate provides the following daily RDA for Vitamin C 48%, Potassium 19%, Vitamin B-6 10%, Magnesium 8%, and Calcium 2%.

Ways to increase pomegranate in your diet...

Eat: pomegranate seeds fresh from the fruit; pomegranate in green salads or fruit salads; guacamole made with pomegranate instead of tomato; pomegranate relish; pomegranate molasses (made without sugar); pomegranate glazed carrots; pomegranate and orange salsa; pomegranate sprinkled on oven roasted vegetables; barley and wild rice with pomegranate seeds; roasted brussel sprouts with pomegranate molasses; pomegranate and honey syrup; pomegranate in yogurt;...

Drink: pomegranate juice (without added sugars, preservatives, and/or other additives);...

* **Prunes (Dried Plums)** - When plums are dried, they become what most people know as prunes. When purchasing packaged prunes, it is good to know that many suppliers, in an effort to better market their product, are changing the name of their product from

prunes to dried plums. The end product is still the same. As with other fruits, the dried or dehydrated version of plums contain a higher concentration of the vitamins and minerals needed for healthy blood pressure. An exception to this higher concentration is that vitamin the C content is higher in a fresh fruit than when it is dried. There are many varieties and colors of plums. Prunes are usually made from the bluish purple European plum that despite its name is grown in temperate regions worldwide. Prunes are sold with or without pits. If you buy prepackaged prunes, make sure that there are no added sugars, preservatives, and/or other additives.

One cup of pitted prunes provides the following daily RDA for Potassium 36%, Vitamin B-6 20%, Magnesium 17%, Calcium 7%, and Vitamin C 1%.

Ways to increase prunes in your diet...

Eat: prunes as a snack straight from package; chopped prunes as a topping in oatmeal; chopped prunes in a nut, grain, fruit, and seed trail mix; (prunes used for cooking can be soaked in water to rehydrate them somewhat and reduce cooking time); stewed prunes with oranges and cinnamon; stewed prunes and dried apricots; stewed prunes, dried figs, and sweet apples;...

Drink: prune juice (without added sugars, preservatives, and/or other additives);...

* **Raisins (Dried Grapes)** - Raisins are dried grapes. Grapes used to make raisins are 55% to 80+% water but when dried their moisture content is less than 19%. Just like described in prunes, except for vitamin C, the dried raisins contain a higher concentration of the vitamins and minerals needed for healthy blood pressure than the same volume of fresh grapes. Raisins are produced around the world but about half of the world's supply of raisins are grown in California. Some sources say raisins were probably discovered by accident in ancient times when sun dried grapes were found on the vines.

One cup of raisins (not packed) provides the following daily RDA for Potassium 31%, Vitamin B-6 15, Magnesium 11%, Calcium 7%, and Vitamin C 5%.

Ways to increase raisins in your diet...

Eat: raisins as a snack straight from package; raisins in green salads, fruit salads, or vegetable salads and slaws; raisins in oatmeal or other hot cereals; raisins in dry cereals; raisins, almonds, and brown rice; raisins as an ingredient in a granola or trail mix; raisins, onion, apple, and baked bean casserole; sautéed raisins and spinach; sautéed raisin, carrot, bell pepper, and onion salad; raisins, red cabbage, and apples casserole; raisin and honey spread; sautéed raisins and winter squash;...

* **Watermelon** - Watermelons grow on long sprawling vines and come in many colors (both the outer rind and the inner flesh). They also come in many sizes and can have seeds or be seedless. Unlike some fruits, all parts of a watermelon are edible, including the seeds and the rind. Each part has nutrients that help with blood pressure control and the watermelon flesh and rind are also a potential diuretic.

One normal serving (about 2 cups or 1 slice) of watermelon provides the following daily RDA for Vitamin C 37%, Potassium 8%, Magnesium 7%, Vitamin B-6 5%, and Calcium 2%.

Ways to increase watermelon in your diet...

Eat: the number one way is fresh watermelon sliced and eaten raw; watermelon in green salads or fruit salads; blended watermelon, cantaloupe, and kiwi soup (serve chilled); watermelon in yogurt; watermelon, peach, and tomato salsa; grilled watermelon slices; watermelon stir-fried with vegetables; cooked watermelon rind and carrot soup; watermelon gummies; watermelon rind, carrot, and pineapple slaw; stir-fry watermelon rind, bell pepper, onion, and garlic; dried or roasted watermelon seeds;...

Drink: watermelon juice (without added sugars, preservatives, and/or other additives);...

Drinking Vegetables and Fruits:

In most cases, eating vegetables and fruits is the best way to get the nutrients you need but it is sometimes hard to get the recommended 4.5 servings of vegetables and fruits a day just by eating. Juicing or blending vegetables and fruits are methods that have been used to easily increase consumption. There is a however a difference between juicing and blending.

A juicer separates the nutrient rich liquid of vegetables and fruits from the fiber or pulp. You must have a juicer to accomplish this process. On the plus side, drinking the liquid juice with no pulp gives a faster release and absorption of nutrients. On the negative side, juicing can be more expensive because the amount of juice that can be obtained relative to the volume of the produce. In addition, since many nutrients are found in the fiber and pulp, juicing does not give you as much of the food's nutrients as using the blending method. The best juicer recipes usually contain one or two juicy components, one leafy green or root component, and one sweet component. These combinations along with other ingredients can also be used in a blender to make smoothies.

A blender is just that. Whatever you put in the blender is what you will get to drink. The volume of this drink will also be higher than obtained from the same amount of vegetables and fruits in a juicer. Blended vegetables with the fiber and pulp retained give a more filling drink and a slower more sustained release of the blended nutrients. This fiber and pulp content also makes you fill fuller which helps reduce overeating and is helpful in the digestive process. The blended drink made in a blender is sometimes called a smoothie. Another plus about making smoothies is that you can also add nuts, seeds, milk, and/or yogurt to increase your intake of calcium and healthy fats. You can also add spices and/or honey to enhance the taste of your smoothie.

Every person's tastes are different, and some find the texture of some blended raw vegetables to be too grainy so try different combinations to find something you like. If you like a drink combination, the more likely you are to make and drink it on a regular basis. One of my favorite blended smoothie drink recipes that I make quite often is to use two overripe bananas, a half a cup of blueberries, a cup of 2% milk, and a half a cup of ice cubes (the ice chills the drink and the water in the ice helps balance out the taste of the ingredients). I also like smoothies made from two sticks of celery, the segments from three oranges (peel and seeds removed), a cup of ice, and a dash of turmeric.

Be sure to wash all fruits and vegetables thoroughly before juicing or blending.

~~~~~~~~~

Beans

Beans have been a great source of protein for thousands of years and are another rich source of needed vitamins and minerals. Beans are also high in protein and used as meat substitutes in many diets and recipes. There are many varieties of beans to choose from and all are great additions to an economical and nutritious diet. As you will see in the RDA values listed below some varieties of beans have a very high mineral content. Beans can be purchased fresh, frozen, canned, or dried. Remember if you buy canned beans, be sure to get low or no sodium brands with no added sugars or preservatives. If your canned beans do contain sodium, it is best to rinse them before using to remove as much of the added sodium as possible. For this book I will list the most common types of beans consumed in America that are highest in the three important minerals needed for effective blood pressure control (potassium, magnesium, and calcium).

* Black Bean

One cup of black beans provides the following daily RDA for Potassium 78%, Magnesium 73%, Calcium 29%, and Vitamin B-6 25%.

* Kidney Bean

One cup of raw kidney beans provides the following daily RDA for Potassium 73%, Magnesium 64%, Vitamin B-6 35%, Calcium 26%, and Vitamin C 13%.

* Pinto Bean

One cup of raw pinto beans provides the following daily RDA for Magnesium 85%, Potassium 76%, Vitamin B-6 45%, Calcium 21%, and Vitamin C 20%.

* Soybean

One cup of raw soybeans provides the following daily RDA for Magnesium 130%, Potassium 95%, Calcium 51%, Vitamin B-6 35%, and Vitamin C 18%.

Ways to increase beans in your diet...

Beans can be cooked ingredients in a multitude of soups, salads, stews, casseroles, or rice dishes; some examples are cooked black beans added to green salads; beans, corn, cucumber, and celery salad; three bean salad; mixed bean soups; dried beans soaked then cooked by boiling to be eaten as a side dish or used in other recipes; black beans and rice; black bean, tomato, and onion salsa; beans in no-salt added chili; burgers made with black, kidney, pinto, or soy beans instead of meat; kidney bean stew; baked beans (without bacon); sautéed soybean, onions, and garlic; dry roasted soybeans as a snack or added to green salads;...

Nuts

Nuts serve as a good source of potassium and magnesium. Some are also a good source of healthy Omega-3 fats. The American Heart Association (for a 2000 calorie a day diet) recommends getting four to five servings of nuts a week (with an average serving of nuts being about 1 ounce). It is important to eat nuts either raw or dry roasted. Never eat nuts or seeds that have been roasted in oils and/or have added salt. Oil roasting in heated hydrogenated oils causes increases in blood pressure. There are many varieties of nuts that provide many health benefits. Nuts provide protein, fiber, healthy unsaturated fats, and heart healthy vitamins and minerals. Nuts are generally high in calories, and some contain Omega-6 fats that are not as healthy unless balanced by the consumption of Omega-3 fats. For these reasons, it is important that you don't go overboard in your daily consumption.

As I did with beans, I will list the most common types of nuts consumed in America and that are highest in the three important minerals needed for effective blood pressure control (potassium, magnesium, and calcium). All the nuts listed are tree nuts. Peanuts are legumes and not a tree nut. Peanuts are also reported to have beneficial nutrients but I did not include the peanut because peanuts have a high level of omega-6 fatty acids and because there is a high prevalence of peanut allergies in today's population.

* Almonds

Known and consumed since ancient times, almonds are thought to have originated in China or central Asia. The almond tree was brought to California from Spain in the 1700's. The only place almonds are grown commercially in North America today is in California. If you use almonds as your daily serving of nuts, the daily amount would be twenty to twenty four almonds.

One ounce (about 23 nuts) of sliced almonds provides the following daily RDA for Magnesium 19%, Calcium 7%, and Potassium 5%.

* Brazil Nut

Brazil nuts come from trees that grow wild in the Amazon rain forest region of South America. If you use Brazil nuts as your daily serving of nuts, the daily amount would be six to eight nuts. Note that a single serving of Brazil nuts provides over 25% of your total daily fat requirement so don't over indulge on this nut. Another reason not to over consume is that Brazil nuts contain selenium that in large quantities can be poisonous. The take away from this is that eating six to eight Brazil nuts a day as your daily nut intake is good but more than that on a daily basis is not.

One ounce of whole Brazil nuts (about 6 nuts) provides the following daily RDA for Magnesium 26%, Potassium 5%, and Calcium 4%.

* Cashews

Cashews originated in Brazil but are now grown in tropical regions around the world. The USA consumes over 90% of all cashew production. If you use cashews as your daily serving of nuts, the daily amount would be sixteen to eighteen nuts.

One ounce of cashews (about 18 nuts) provides the following daily RDA for Magnesium 20%, Vitamin B-6 5%, Potassium 5%, and Calcium 1%.

* Pistachio

Pistachios grow on flowering nut trees and have been around since prehistoric times. Humans have been eating pistachios for at least 9,000 years. Almost all of the pistachios produced in the United States are grown in California. If you use pistachios as your daily serving of nuts, the daily amount would be forty seven to forty nine nuts.

One ounce of pistachios (about 49 nuts) provides the following daily RDA for Vitamin B-6 25%, Magnesium 8%, Potassium 8%, Calcium 3%, and Vitamin C 2%.

* Walnuts

Walnuts are another nut that humans have been eating since prehistoric times. Like pistachios, the majority of the walnuts grown commercially in the United States are grown in California. There are several varieties of walnuts. Even though the black walnut is native to the United States, the most widely consumed is the English walnut which has a milder taste. The English walnut originally came from Persia and the tree was imported and established in California in the 1700's.

If you use walnuts as your daily serving of nuts, the daily amount would be thirteen to fifteen nut halves.

One oz of halved walnuts (about 14 halves) provides the following daily RDA for Magnesium 11%, Vitamin B-6 10%, Potassium 3%, and Calcium 2%.

Ways to increase nuts in your diet...

Since the recommended daily serving amounts are small, most nuts are eaten raw as snacks; dry roasted (without salt); added to salads; added to stir-fries; added to yogurt; as an ingredient in granola or trail mix; made into butter spreads (without additives); kale chips with almond butter; oven toasted spiced nuts;...

~~~~~~~~~

Fish

Fatty Fish – Wild Salmon, Mackerel, Herring, Lake Trout, Sardines, Tuna

Fish is also a recommended food choice for heart health and blood pressure control. The American Heart Association recommends eating at least two 3.5 ounce servings of fish a week. Fish are low in calories, a good source of protein, low in unhealthy saturated fat, and a good source of healthy omega-3 fatty acids. Omega-3 fatty acids reduce inflammation in the body that can damage blood vessels and the heart. Omega-3 fatty acids also appear to reduce the risk of sudden cardiac death. Fatty fish such as wild salmon, mackerel, herring, lake trout, sardines, and tuna have higher levels of Omega-3 and vitamin D. Vitamin D is needed for the body to absorb calcium effectively. These types of fish are the best choices for a diet with blood pressure reduction and maintenance as a priority. Also, these fish (either fresh or frozen) that are wild caught (not farmed) are less likely to contain high levels of mercury and higher levels of omega-3 fatty acids.

How you prepare these fish is as important as the type of fish. Deep frying fish in oil cancels any health benefits you would receive from eating fish (or any other food for that matter). Each of these fish has distinctive flavors so try several and find the methods of cooking and recipes you like. Having a variety of dishes to choose from will make it easier to incorporate fish into your normal weekly diet.

Ways to increase fish in your diet...

Fish can be eaten poached, baked, grilled, or microwaved; use lemon juice, spices and/or herbs to enhance flavors; fish fillet soup; grilled fish and vegetables; foil baked fish and vegetables; foil baked fish, oranges, lemon, and chives;...

~~~~~~~~~

Dairy

* Milk – Low fat 2%, 1%, or Fat-free

Dairy farms in the United States produce about twenty one 21 billion gallons of milk a year. Milk is another food that has been consumed by humans since prehistoric times. Milk from cows provides a major source for calcium, and most milk in the United States is fortified with vitamin D. These two nutrients work together in reducing blood pressure. The American Heart Association recommends consuming 2 to 3 cups of milk or yogurt every day.

One cup of milk provides the following daily RDA for Calcium 29%, Potassium 9%, Magnesium 6%, Vitamin B-6 5%, and Sodium 4%. Note, if milk is fortified with vitamin D (and about 98% of milk sold in the United States is) then a cup of this milk also has an RDA for vitamin D 50%.

* Yogurt – non-fat

Yogurt is produced by the bacterial fermentation of milk. Because many of the pre-packaged yogurts contain added sugars and other additives, and the fact that many do not add vitamin D, I would not recommend pre-packaged yogurts unless you are certain that no unhealthy ingredients have been added. If you make your own yogurt from fresh milk, it should contain the same vitamins and minerals as found in the milk.

Three fourths cup of yogurt (one standard size container) provides the following daily RDA for Calcium 18%, Potassium 6%, Vitamin B-6 5%, Magnesium 4%, and Sodium 2%.

Ways to increase milk or yogurt in your diet...

Milk: the most common way to consume milk is to drink it; use milk as an ingredient in soups; make fresh cottage cheese; add to a bowl of granola; pour on top of a bowl of cooked oatmeal; make yogurt; add it to hot herbal teas; use milk as an ingredient in blended smoothies; make smoothie popsicles; eat yogurt plain or with fruit and/or nut toppings; use yogurt as an ingredient in blended smoothies; yogurt can be substituted for sour cream in many recipes;...

~~~~~~~~~

Herbs and Spice

Herbs and spices are added to all sorts of recipes to enhance the flavor of foods and to make eating more pleasurable. Many of them also are used for their medicinal properties. The familiar herbs and spices I have listed below all can have beneficial effects in maintaining a healthy blood pressure level.

* Basil

There are three main types of basil: sweet, purple, and bush. Within these types are more 60 varieties with subtle flavor differences (such as sweet basil, lemon basil, lime basil, cinnamon basil, clove basil, and more).

One tablespoon of ground basil provides the following daily RDA for Calcium 10%, Magnesium 8%, Vitamin B-6 5%, and Potassium 3%.

* Black Pepper

The fruit of the black pepper plant which when dried is called a peppercorn. This peppercorn is then ground into the more familiar form of black pepper. Black pepper is a good anti-inflammatory agent. Piperine is the substance that gives black pepper its taste. This piperine is known to increase the bioavailability of many nutritional substances. One of these is curcumin, a compound in turmeric that promotes healthy blood circulation. Another is increased absorption of Coenzyme Q10 (CoQ10).

One tablespoon of ground black pepper provides the following daily RDA for Calcium 3%, Magnesium 3%, and Potassium 2%.

* Ginger

The spice ginger comes from the underground stem of the flowering ginger plant. Ginger is used as a spicy and aromatic ingredient in many Asian recipes and has been used for its medicinal properties in many cultures for centuries. Ginger acts as a blood thinner, inhibits the formation of inflammatory compounds, and has direct anti-inflammatory effects.

One tablespoon of ground ginger provides the following daily RDA for Magnesium 2%, and Potassium 1%.

* Oregano

Oregano is used in many Mediterranean and Mexican recipes. It is an herb that has also been used in cooking and for medicinal purposes for thousands of years. Oregano has forty two times more antioxidants than apples and twelve times more antioxidants than oranges. What makes oregano very effective against high blood pressure is a compound known as carvacrol. Carvacrol has been shown to reduce average arterial pressure and it also helps controlling heart rate.

One teaspoon of dried oregano provides the following daily RDA for Calcium 2%, and Magnesium 1%.

* Turmeric

Turmeric is a member of the ginger plant family. The dried powered spice used in many recipes comes from the root of the turmeric plant. Turmeric is native to India and Southeast Asia. It has been used to flavor food and as an herbal medicine for several thousand years. The curcumin in turmeric reduces inflammation and improves the regulation of blood pressure. As noted in the black pepper section above, when coupled with black pepper, curcumin is more readily absorbed by the body.

One tablespoon of ground turmeric provides the following daily RDA for Vitamin B-6 5%, Potassium 4%, Magnesium 3%, Vitamin C 3%, and Calcium 1%.

~~~~~~~~~~

Supplements

Dietary supplements may be sold in a variety of forms, including tablets, capsules, powders, chewables, or liquids. They may be standalone supplements or mixed with other nutrients or ingredients. The best way to get the nutrients you need to maintain healthy blood pressure levels is to consume them from their natural state.

Unlike for foods, the FDA does not have the authority to review dietary supplement products for safety and effectiveness before they are marketed. Because of this, exercise caution if you decide to take a supplement for any of the vitamins, minerals, or compounds that have been discussed. Before you take a dietary supplement, be sure to carefully read the Supplement Facts panel and labels on the supplement package.

If you decide to take the supplement, you should heed and follow any precautions listed on the label. Also be aware of how the supplement may react with other supplements or medicines you may take. Consuming supplements in too high amounts may create an imbalance in other nutrients and may even be toxic. Be aware of the possibility of unexpected side effects from taking any supplement. If you are taking any kind of prescription medication, always discuss with your healthcare provider about any possible interactions a supplement might have with that medication.

The list below looks at each of the important nutrients identified in this chapter, and some of the pros and cons for taking supplements for these nutrients:

* Calcium

The most common calcium supplements contain either calcium carbonate or calcium citrate. Calcium helps blood vessels tighten and relax when they need to. Healthy blood pressure levels depend on balanced ratios of magnesium to calcium.

My recommendation is that you should try to get your needed calcium from dietary sources such as leafy greens, milk, and if you are lactose intolerant, from healthy calcium fortified food and drinks.

Calcium supplements taken without an adequate and offsetting amount of magnesium may cause damage to the heart and blood vessels. Calcium supplements have been shown to interact with many different prescription medicines, including blood pressure medications. Excess calcium over time can actually cause damage to your circulatory system that will lead to an increase in blood pressure. Excess calcium may also contribute to the development of kidney stones. Some calcium supplements may cause effects such as gas, constipation, or bloating. So again, I do not recommend taking calcium supplements.

* Coenzyme Q10 (CoQ10)

CoQ10 is a fat-soluble, vitamin-like substance that is naturally produced in the human body and functions like an antioxidant. Healthy food sources for CoQ10 include leafy green vegetables and fatty fish. As we age, the amount we produce decreases and a supplement is a good choice to increase the amount of this nutrient in our body. The recommended supplement amount for adults is between 30 to 200 milligrams daily depending your age and on how much you are getting in your normal diet.

These supplements should be taken with a meal. CoQ10 is fat-soluble and to be absorbed effectively it must be eaten with meal containing fats (healthy fats). Although in most cases they are mild and improve within a few days, some possible side effects from CoQ10 supplements may include fatigue, flu-like symptoms, heartburn, insomnia, irritability, itching, nausea, or sensitivity to light. This is one of the supplements that I would recommend, especially if you are over 60. From the information I gained during my research, I personally decided to start taking CoQ10 supplements and did not experience any of these side effects. I take two 100 mg soft gels daily and have seen improvements in my energy levels and a reduction in blood pressure. The brand I take also has piperine (from black pepper) as an additive that helps enhance absorption and bioavailability of the CoQ10.

* Magnesium

Magnesium is an essential mineral for many systems in the body. It is the fourth most abundant mineral in the human body. The daily RDA for magnesium is 320 mg for women and 420 mg for men, an amount that is not being achieved by most Americans. Magnesium affects blood pressure by increasing the ability of the smooth muscle cells in the blood vessels to relax. Magnesium deficiency increases with age and it is estimated that as many of 75% of people in the United States have a magnesium deficiency. As stated in the calcium supplement section, healthy blood pressure levels depend on a balanced ratio of magnesium to calcium. Magnesium is also needed for vitamin D production and functions in the body. If you have a muscle spasm (charlie horse) when your stretch your legs, you may have a magnesium deficiency.

Magnesium supplements have few risks and many healthcare professionals recommend that adults take supplements on a regular basis. On note of caution, don't take magnesium supplements if you have kidney problems. Some possible side effects for some from taking too much magnesium supplement may be upset stomach, nausea, and diarrhea. If you are not getting enough magnesium from your diet, I would recommend taking a magnesium supplement.

One of first supplements I started taking just after I started my research on natural ways to reduce and control my blood pressure levels was magnesium. As with the CoQ10 supplement, I have not experienced any negative side effects. I started taking two 100 mg tablets per day and began to see immediate improvements in my average blood pressure readings. The brand I take is chelated which optimizes bioavailability. When minerals in supplements are chelated, more of the mineral will be absorbed in the intestinal tract than a mineral supplement that is non-chelated.

* Omega-3 Fatty Acids

Omega-3 fatty acids are considered essential fatty acids necessary for human health. Omega-3 fatty acids are not produced in the body, they can only be gotten through dietary sources. You should try to get your needed omega-3 from dietary sources such as fatty fish, walnuts, leafy green vegetables, squash, soybeans, strawberries, milk, and eggs. Remember that you can get your RDA of omega-3 by eating two 3.5 ounce servings of fish a week (less than 1/2 pound per week). Even less if you eat some of the other foods containing this nutrient.

The FDA has ruled that omega-3 fatty acids supplements are safe and lawful, as long as daily amount taken does not exceed three grams per person a day from the combination of food and supplement sources. The potential side effects, precautions, and risks associated with taking too much omega-3 supplement are many. A report from the Mayo Clinic on the side effects of

omega-3 said "Omega-3 may also cause abnormal heart rhythm, abnormally high urination, acid reflux, anemia, anorexia, bad breath, bad taste in the mouth, bloating, bloody urine, blurred vision, burping, cancer, changes in energy and physical activity (in infants whose mothers received supplementation), changes in homocysteine levels, the common cold, constipation, diarrhea, dizziness, excess fat in the stool, fainting (in pregnant women at birth), a feeling of ants crawling on the skin, a feeling of burning or prickling, a feeling of lifelessness, fever, fishy hiccups, gas, headache, heart attack, hospitalization (chest pain, congestive heart failure, or nervous system problems), increased risk of stroke, indigestion, intolerance to capsule number or size, mania, memory problems, muscle pain or swelling, nausea, the need for surgery (coronary revascularization), nervous system toxicity, nosebleed, restlessness, sleep problems, sudden cardiac death, skin problems (irritation, itching, rashes), stomach pain, throat pain, tiredness, vomiting, and weight gain."

Studies show that fish rich in omega-3 fatty acids should be a part of a heart healthy diet yet there is growing concern about the levels of mercury in fish. On the other hand, studies on omega-3 supplements have not shown proof of having the same effectiveness as eating fish. The science on the effectiveness and proper dose of omega-3 supplements still does not seem to be conclusive. Weighing the risks of the supplements against the possibility of getting to much mercury from fish, and the availability of omega-3 in other foods, I would still recommend getting your omega-3 fatty acids from consuming the foods that contain it.

* Potassium

Potassium is important in controlling blood pressure by helping balance out the negative effects of sodium (salt). Having a high sodium/low potassium level reduces the ability of your kidneys to remove the excess salt. Potassium also plays an important role in many other body functions like various chemical reactions, nerve signal transmissions, fluid balance, and muscle contractions.

You can get all the potassium your body needs just by eating a healthy diet. Many vegetables, fruits, beans, and nuts contain good amounts of potassium and there are no reports of negative effects in healthy people from potassium obtained through dietary intake.

There are risks of getting too much potassium by taking supplements and your kidney's can have a difficult time flushing excess potassium if you exceed your body's need for it. Some of the medications prescribed for high blood pressure taken along with potassium supplements may cause high levels of potassium in the blood. High levels of potassium are unsafe. The effects of too much potassium in the blood could be weakness, uneven heartbeat, mental confusion, stomach pain, numbness or tingling feelings, low blood pressure, and death.

Because you can get all the potassium you need by eating a healthy diet, my recommendation is that you should never take potassium supplements unless you are instructed to do so by your doctor.

* Vitamin B-6

Vitamin B-6 is naturally present in many foods and people who have diets high in vitamin B-6 foods have lower overall rates of heart disease. Vitamin B-6 helps control blood pressure by controlling homocysteine levels in the blood. Homocysteine is produced when red meat and dairy products are broken down in the body, and high levels of homocysteine give an increased risk of heart attacks and strokes. Fish, starchy vegetables, and fruits (other than citrus) are all good sources for vitamin B-6.

Most people in the United States get enough vitamin B-6 from foods in their diet. The average daily recommended amount for young adults is 1.3mg, for women ages 51 and older - 1.5mg, and for men ages 51 and older - 1.7mg. The current recommended maximum daily intake is 100 mg. Most of the over the counter vitamin B-6 supplements have 25mg to 100mg per tablet or capsule. 100mg is more than 50 times the daily recommended amount which would make it very easy to take more than the daily recommended maximum.

People almost never get too much vitamin B6 from food but you can experience side effects from taking high levels of vitamin B-6 in supplements. High levels over time can be toxic and cause severe nerve damage and loss of control of bodily movements. Other side effects of too much vitamin B-6 may include sensitivity to sunlight, painful skin patches, numbness, heartburn, and/or nausea. If you feel that you need to take a supplement for B-6, then you could try a multi-vitamin that would have 3mg to 6mg per tablet. While more than needed in a day, it is a much lower amount of B-6 than you would get in a standalone supplement for it. Because of its availability in a healthy diet, I would not recommend taking supplements for vitamin B-6.

* Vitamin C

Vitamin C acts as a diuretic that helps remove sodium and water from the body which in turn helps relax blood vessel walls and decrease blood pressure. The average daily recommended amount for adult women is 75mg and for adult men is 90mg. Vitamin C is also known as ascorbic acid. Because it is a water-soluble nutrient and destroyed by heat, it is best to get your daily requirement from raw vegetables and fruits.

Studies have shown that vitamin C supplements do not provide the same protective benefits as getting vitamin C from dietary sources such as an orange or drinking orange juice. Normally, the body can only use about 200mg to 250mg of vitamin C a day with any excess being expelled through urine. The recommended maximum daily intake of vitamin C for adults is 2000 mg. Daily ingestion of amounts greater than this may contribute to kidney stone formation and/or cause diarrhea, fatigue, insomnia, rashes, gastritis, and/or nausea. Frequent use of chewable vitamin C supplements may cause dental erosion. With many of the today's vitamin C supplements offered with a 1000mg content as well as packages of chewable or dissolving lozenge, it is very easy to exceed the maximum intake level.

During the time I was on a mostly convenience food diet and before I had done the research on blood pressure control, I was taking a 1000mg vitamin C supplement pretty much daily. After doing this research and switching to a more healthy diet, I realized that I no longer needed to take these supplements and seeing the potential side effects, I stopped taking them. As I said in the review for vitamin B-6 above, if you feel that you are not getting enough vitamin C in your diet and need to take a supplement, then choose a multivitamin that contains vitamin C in the 60mg to 90mg range. Because of its availability in a healthy diet, the fact that a normal excess would be excreted through the urine, and the potential side effects of taking amounts over the maximum intake levels, I would not recommend taking supplements for vitamin C.

* Vitamin D

Vitamin D is called the "sunshine" vitamin. Vitamin D acts similar to ACE inhibitors in reducing high blood pressure and studies have shown that people with low levels of vitamin D are more likely to have high blood pressure. Vitamin D is needed for the absorption of calcium in the stomach and for calcium functions in the body. Vitamin D is also an anti-inflammatory. A deficiency of vitamin D can cause increased vascular resistance, which leads to increased blood pressure.

The human body can get the vitamin D it needs by the exposure of bare skin to sunlight (specifically ultraviolet B). The vitamin D produced during exposure to sunlight is stored in fatty cells in the body and released when the sunlight is not available. It is estimated that with full body exposure to the sun, a fair-skinned person can produce up to 20,000 IU of vitamin D3 in 20 minutes. This is stored in body fat and then released when the sunlight is gone. Unfortunately, the half-life of this vitamin D is only two weeks which means it will be depleted quickly in times when exposure to sunlight is limited. Studies conducted recently say that up to 50% of the world's population is deficient in vitamin D. Some of the reasons for this are that most foods that contain vitamin D have only small amounts, more people are staying inside or covering up and/or wearing sunscreen when outside to reduce skin cancer risks, production of vitamin D gets less as we age, and more people are living in latitudes further away from the equator.

Most of the people in the United States do not get enough vitamin D. Most of their dietary intake of vitamin D comes from "fortified" foods such as milk, some orange juice, some cereals, and other foods with added vitamin D.

For vitamin D, the average daily recommended amount for adults under 70 is 600 IU, for those 70+ it is 800 IU. The recommended maximum daily intake of vitamin D is 4000 IU. Taking supplements in daily amounts greater than 4000 IU over a period of time can cause excessively high levels of calcium in the blood and lower magnesium amounts in the body. Side effects from taking vitamin D are not commonly experienced unless too much is taken.

Because of the facts above showing why most people are not getting enough vitamin D, many different sources recommend taking a 1000 IU supplement of vitamin D on a daily basis. There are two types of vitamin D supplements, D2 derived from plants, and D3 derived from animals. Research has shown that the human body utilizes vitamin D3 better.

Vitamin D3 is another supplement I would recommend to those interested in having healthy blood pressure levels. I spend a good bit of time outside in the sun gardening and hobby farming but I still take a 1000 IU supplement of vitamin D3 every day.

Summary: recommendations for taking supplements:

Potassium - **No** supplementation - get potassium from dietary sources

Magnesium - **Yes** - 200 mg per day

Calcium - **No** supplementation - get calcium from dietary sources

Coenzyme Q10 (CoQ10) - **Yes** - 200 mg per day

Omega-3 fatty acids - **No** - get Omega-3 from dietary sources

Vitamin B-6 - **Maybe** - only at low dose in multi-vitamin supplement with no more than 6 mg per day

Vitamin C - **Maybe** - only at low dose in multi-vitamin supplement with no more than 90 mg per day

Vitamin D - **Yes** - 1000 IU per day of D3

Caution on multivitamins and/or other supplements: Avoid taking more than one multivitamin product at the same time, avoid taking multivitamins that have the same nutrient as a supplement being taken, avoid taking multivitamins or supplements while eating fortified foods that have the same nutrient(s) as those being taken. These combinations could result in going over the maximum daily intake limits on some nutrients and result in serious consequences.

~~~~~~~~

Other

I am listing items in this section that did not exactly fit in any of the above categories but are items that I personally am using in my effort to reduce and maintain a healthy blood pressure level.

* Hibiscus Tea

Hibiscus tea has been very popular in Africa and Mexico for thousands of years. Hibiscus is a flower plant with a variety of health benefits. According to many clinical human studies (these studies are linked below), hibiscus tea can lower blood pressure and speed up your metabolism, and it also has anti-inflammatory effects. Hibiscus has a very high antioxidant content (multiple times higher than green tea).

I had a serious coffee habit and was drinking several cups of coffee throughout the day and evening. I was looking for something to replace this habit when my research pointed to Hibiscus tea. I liked hot tea and hibiscus tea looked like something I could use to cut back or replace my habit of drinking caffeinated coffee. Once I tried it, I found that I liked hibiscus tea enough to drink it instead of a cup of coffee. I also make an ice tea from hibiscus. I make it about a gallon at a time with added sliced lemons and sometimes sweeten it with orange blossom honey. I keep it in the refrigerator and drink it with meals and whenever I get an urge to have a sugary carbonated soft drink.

* Lemons

Lemons help lower blood pressure by removing rigidity in blood vessels keeping them pliable and soft. Lemons are a citrus fruit high in vitamin C which is a powerful anti oxidant. One lemon provides the following daily RDA for Vitamin C 51%, Potassium 2%, Calcium 1%, and Magnesium 1%. Lemon peel serves as a flavorful spice and lemon juice is used in many recipes to enhance the flavors of the other ingredients and reduce the need to add salt for flavor. Adding lemon juice makes plain water more palatable.

This was another item I started to use to cut back on my coffee habit. Instead of having a cup of coffee first thing in the morning, I started drinking a cup of hot boiled water mixed with the juice of one lemon and a spoonful of honey. This alternative is much more heart healthy than coffee. I was amazed that I got a better, more sustained, and longer lasting boost from this than I ever got from a hot cup of caffeinated coffee.

* Olive Oil

I added this final item because during my research for heart healthy recipes, I found many suggested stir-fry recipes for vegetables. Unfortunately, I found that the vegetable oil I was using was actually negating all the benefits of the vegetables I was beginning to cook this way. With further research, I found that olive oil is most healthy option when stir-frying or sautéing foods.

Olive oil contains omega-3 fatty acids like those found in fish. Omega-3 fatty acids not produced in the body but are considered essential fatty acids necessary for human health. According to the University of Maryland Medical Center, Omega-3 fatty acids help lower the risk of heart disease and other ailments. The fat content of olive oil is 74 percent monosaturated fat, 14 percent of saturated fat, and 12 percent of polysaturated fat. To stir-fry or sauté vegetables, choose extra light olive oil because it has a high smoke point (over 460 degrees Fahrenheit). See more about the importance of the smoke point in oils in the "Things To Avoid" section in this book.

"Let food be thy medicine and medicine be thy food." ~ Hippocrates

~~~~~~~~~

B: Exercise

Exercise is just as important as diet when it comes to preventing or reducing high blood pressure. Think of it this way, if you want to be able to run 10 miles you start out with an exercise plan. You start by running, but you can only run for a short distance until you get tired. You continue with your plan, and after a while as your muscles strengthen, you are able to run further with less effort, and over time, you reach your goal. Your heart is a muscle and it too will grow stronger as you exercise. As your heart muscle grows stronger, it takes less effort for it to pump blood and lowers how much force it exerts on your blood vessels (lowered blood pressure).

As a society, we have adopted increasingly sedentary lifestyles. It may take more effort to get up and get moving but if you want to keep your blood pressure in check or if you already have high blood pressure, physical exercise is essential for keeping your heart strong, promoting circulation, and for keeping your blood pressure under control. If you are currently inactive, start slow with any new exercise routine. If you are currently being medically treated for any condition, check with your doctor first before starting any new exercise programs.

The American Heart Association states that these activities are especially beneficial for the heart when done regularly: Brisk walking, hiking, stair-climbing, jogging, running, bicycling, rowing or swimming, fitness classes at your appropriate level, activities such team sports, a dance class, or fitness games.

If you are not active today, gradually work up to a moderate activity routine. It is absolutely OK if it takes a few weeks for you to get up to your target activity schedule. Your target should be for a moderate exercise activity for at least 30 minutes a day, and at least 5 days a week. This can be in one 30-minute block, or it can be broken down into two 15-minute sessions, or three 10-minute sessions as long as you get 30 minutes total exercise in a day. Once you are comfortable with completing moderate exercise on a regular basis and you find you are short on time, you can get the same benefits by doing a vigorous activity (like jogging) for 20 minutes a day, 3 to 4 days a week.

In addition to the traditional exercise activities, you can also use these methods to help achieve your moderate daily exercise goals:

* Put the laundry away a few items at a time rather than all at once.

* Carry groceries from the car into your home one bag or package at a time.

* Mow the lawn. If you use a riding mower, give it up and use a walk behind. Even if it the walk behind is self-propelled the walking will give you exercise.

* Rake the leaves with a rake. Not a blower or riding mower vacuum.

* Start and tend to a garden.

* Park farther away from where you work or where you shop and walk briskly to your destination.

* Take your child or grandchild for a brisk walk.

* Play kick the can with your child, grandchild, or friends.

* Play with a hula-hoop or jump rope.

* Your phone does not glue you to your seat, walk in place or pace in your office while you are talking.

* Instead of using the phone or email, walk down the hall to talk to a colleague.

* If you work at a desk or you sit for long periods of time at your job, take a brisk 10-minute walk during your lunch break.

* Avoid the elevator, take the stairs, or walk up or down the escalator.

* Take dancing lessons.

* Exercise while watching TV.

* Hand wash and wax your car.

* If you live in an urban area, walk or bike to the corner store instead of driving.

* Take a 30-minute mall walk with friends.

A side benefit of many of these activities is that it gets you outside into the sunlight. Remember that sunlight is a major source for getting the Vitamin D that you need.

If you want to maintain a healthy blood pressure or to lower a too high pressure, you must get up and exercise. The Mayo Clinic says that for some people, getting some exercise is enough to reduce the need for blood pressure medication. They also say it takes about one to three months for regular exercise to have an impact on your blood pressure and the benefits last only as long as you continue to exercise.

"The key is taking responsibility and initiative, deciding what your life is about and prioritizing your life around the most important things." ~ Stephen Covey

~~~~~~~~

C: Stress Reduction

Stress Reduction

Stress reduction coping methods are one of the most difficult things people with high blood pressure must learn. You get caught up in day-to-day activities that cause you to stress and it is hard to step back and apply some of the techniques that are proven to reduce or counteract that stress.

Stress itself has not been proven to cause chronic high blood pressure but some of the ways we cope with stress like letting it interfere with normal sleep, overeating, drinking alcohol, and other behaviors definitely have an effect on blood pressure. Stress may lead to depression, which in turn may cause self-destructive behavior like smoking, eating unhealthy foods, use of illegal drugs, abusing or not taking prescribed medications all of which can result in higher blood pressure levels.

"One way to get high blood pressure is to go mountain climbing over molehills." ~ Earl Wilson

Many prescription drugs are currently available and being prescribed for dealing with stress but the following natural methods may prove to be just as effective without the associated costs and possible side effects of these drugs.

* **Relax** - Relaxing is important to proper control of blood pressure. Meditation, deep breathing exercises, and yoga all are proven stress reducing activities.

* **Exercise** - Believe it or not, exercise and physical activity are a good ways to relax. See the section on Exercise for ideas on increasing physical activity

* **Simplify** - Eliminate time consuming activities that are not important to you - learn to say no.

* **Go outside** - Not only does it increase the production of Vitamin D in the body, studies have shown that going for a walk outside and communing with nature with provides a positive relaxing health effect. Gardening has shown to have the same effect. Just be sure and turn off your mobile phone if you are walking to relax.

* **Breathe** - Nitric oxide can open constricted blood vessels which lowers blood pressure. You can increase nitric oxide in your blood by closing off one nostril and your mouth then breathing in and out slowly and deeply through one nostril. Concentrating on this activity for a few minutes not increases nitric oxide, it is also can be a meditatively way of relaxing. Deep breathing exercises slow the heart and reduces blood pressure.

* **Keep calm** - Learn to let go. A favorite saying of mine is that "a hundred years from now, none of this is going to make any difference to me one way or another". Learn your stress triggers and avoid those situations if you can. Stressing out about being in a

situation doesn't help because you're already in it. Most of the things you find stressful today will probably not be important to you at all next week. Learn to accept things that you cannot change and move on.

* **Meditation** - A few minutes of meditation a day helps reduce anxiety. To meditate just chose a quiet spot, sit up straight, close your eyes, breath naturally, focus only on your breathing, do no focus on any distracting thoughts just let them float by and gently return your focus back to your breathing. Start by setting a few minutes each day working up to 10 to 20-minute sessions.

* **Unplug** - Turn off your phone and email access. Find an activity you enjoy, read a book or magazine, listen to music, work a puzzle, play a game, or take a nap. Leave work at work.

* **Sleep** - Allow adequate time for sleep in your daily schedule (most folks need 7 to 9 hours of sleep per day to remain healthy). This sounds simple but many of us plan work or activities that take so much time that there is not enough time left in our day for needed sleep time. Relax, slow things down, dim the lights, and decrease stimulation at least 1 hour before bedtime. Sleep in a pitch-black room, cover or hide all the intrusive, annoying lights on electronic devices, TVs, and clocks. If you have outside light coming into your room, use light-blocking curtains to keep your room dark. If you find it helpful to cover outside noises use a fan or white noise machine. Try to stick to a schedule and go to bed at the same time every night even on the days you do not have to work. To relax, try a hot cup of caffeine free herbal tea before bedtime.

" *Believe you can and you're halfway there.*" ~ *Theodore Roosevelt*

~~~~~~~~~~~~

D: Things To Avoid

Things to avoid can be the hardest to accomplish of all the categories in Natural Blood Pressure Control. Habits are our lives on autopilot and they are things we do without giving them much thought. To break a habit you must first admit that you have it and then make a conscious effort stop and make lasting changes. Many of the bad habits we develop that contribute to high blood pressure came as a way to cope with day-to-day stresses we experienced.

"It is easier to prevent bad habits than to break them."
~ Benjamin Franklin

Make sure to replace your old harmful habits with new activities you enjoy. Soon your new activities will become your new habits and will remain when your autopilot takes over. If you have habits or overindulge in some of the items listed below start now to quit or reduce them. For some of the things on this list you may need help from friends or a support group. In some cases, you may even want to consult with a health professional about ways to get advice on where to start.

Things To Avoid If You Want To Reduce And Control High Blood Pressure:

* Alcohol

Drinking too much alcohol can cause high blood pressure. The American Heart Association's recommendation is to limit alcohol consumption to no more than two drinks per day for men and no more than one drink per day for women. Alcohol also contains calories and excessive drinking contributes to unwanted weight gain which is another factor that can cause high blood pressure. If you are a heavy drinker now you should slowly reduce the amount you drink over a two-week span of time. Stopping suddenly creates the risk of developing severe high blood pressure that could last for several days as well as other severe withdrawal symptoms.

* Cigarettes

In addition to cigarettes, avoid secondhand smoke and any form of tobacco. The nicotine in a cigarette raises your blood pressure, and narrows and hardens the walls of your arteries. It also makes your blood more likely to clot. These factors place stresses on your heart and may lead to a heart attack or stroke. Most smokers are both physically and psychologically addicted to cigarettes, which makes it a very hard habit to quit. If you smoke or use tobacco in any form, you may need professional help in order to successfully stop.

* Convenience Foods

Many commercially prepared "Convenience" foods have a high sodium, added sugars, and/or trans-fat content. Foods such as frozen pizza, frozen dinners, processed meats, instant or flavored rice, instant potatoes, boxed dry cereal mixes, instant oatmeal or cereal; pickled products, ramen noodles (especially the flavor package), salad dressings, taco mixes, salted snack foods, and many more highly processed ready to eat convenience foods usually have one or more of unhealthy levels of these added ingredients. Whenever they are available, read the Nutrition Facts labels on these items to see which and how much additives are in the product.

* Over The Counter Medications

To make sure any over the counter (OTC) medication you might buy does not contain ingredients that could cause an increase in your blood pressure, read the medication labels before you buy. The following OTC medications are known to cause increased blood pressure:

- Decongestants that contain pseudoephedrine.

- Non-steroidal Anti-inflammatory Drugs (NSAIDs) pain medications that include naproxen sodium or ibuprofen.

- Some cold and flu medicines may contain these decongestants and NSAIDs.

- Some antacids and other stomach medicines that have a high sodium content.

- Over the counter appetite suppressants.

- Over the counter medicines containing sodium or salt

* Pan or Deep Fried Foods

A study conducted by the Harvard School of Public Health found that people who ate fried food at least once per week had a greater risk for heart disease. They also found that increased frequency of consumption greatly increased the risk.

Any oil that is heated past its smoke point starts to oxidize, breaking down and releasing free radicals. This oxidation of oils from heating leads to increased blood pressure levels. Any heating (and especially deep-frying) will oxidize oils. Even worse is eating restaurant food fried in artificial oils containing trans-fats. When the oil is used multiple times (like in deep fat fryers), it continues to be further degraded and more of it is absorbed into the food being cooked. The lower the smoke point of the oil being used, the more oxidative degradation, and the higher the health risks from eating foods cooked in that oil.

Frying foods also adds a lot of calories and fat to the food being cooked. Eating a lot of fried foods contributes to obesity and being overweight puts you at a higher risk for having high blood pressure.

* Salt (Sodium)

Too much salt (sodium) consumption causes your body holds extra water to flush the salt from your body. This may cause blood pressure to rise because the added water volume puts stress on the heart and blood vessels. Most of the salt you consume does not come from the salt you may add to foods you prepare yourself. In 2016, the FDA stated: "About 75% of dietary sodium comes from eating packaged and restaurant foods. Most Americans eat too much sodium, and too much sodium can raise blood pressure – which can have serious health consequences if not treated."

The body does require a small amount of sodium to function properly but that amount is less than 1/4 teaspoon (575 mg) per day. The recommendation from the American Heart Association is to limit daily sodium intake at no more than 1,500 milligrams. This is about two thirds of a teaspoon of salt. These guidelines are greatly exceeded daily by most people. For a natural method of control, find spices and herbs you like and use them in foods you prepare instead of salt to flavor foods. For processed and purchased foods be sure to check available Nutrition Facts labels and if possible only select foods that contain less than 5% of the daily DRV (dietary reference values). Also, be sure to check the serving size listed as containing that amount. Sometimes the serving size is much less than what will be consumed. If you eat twice as much as the listed serving size, then you have doubled the amount of the listed ingredient. An example, the most common serving size on sliced bread is one slice. How many people make a sandwich with one piece of bread? That means that if one slice which typically has 5% to 7% DRV of salt, then if you use two slices to you are up to 10% to 14% of your salt intake limit.

You do not have to keep an exact record of how much salt you eat, the goal is to reduce the amount of salt you eat as low as possible. Be aware of the salt content of the foods you eat, and always try to eat the foods with the lowest salt level. Look for the words sodium or the symbol Na on nutrition labels and ingredient lists. Also, look at the label for added ingredients that contain sodium. Examples of these would include baking soda, baking powder, disodium phosphate, monosodium glutamate (MSG), sodium alginate, sodium benzoate, sodium bicarbonate, sodium hydroxide, sodium nitrite, sodium propionate, and sodium sulfite.

* Sugar

The simplest reason you should avoid foods and drinks with added sugars is that sugar contributes to obesity that may lead to high blood pressure. The more of your daily calories that come from added sugar, the more you increase the chances of having high blood pressure. Most of the daily sugar intake of Americans comes from the high fructose corn syrup (a man made sweetener) that is added to thousands of processed foods and soft drinks. A lesser amount comes from sucrose (from sugar cane and sugar beets) in the form of table sugar. High sugar content equates to higher calorie levels, which leads people of all ages to be overweight or obese, and as a result potentially higher blood pressure levels. Fructose metabolism creates uric acid as a byproduct within minutes of being ingested. Uric acid suppresses nitric oxide which leads to high blood pressure. Nitric oxide helps your vessels maintain their elasticity. Excess uric acid can also contribute to the formation of kidney stones.

* Solid Fats - Saturated and Trans-fats

Your body needs some fat to function normally in processing fat-soluble vitamins (like A, D, E and K) and essential fatty acids (like Omega-3 and Omega-6). You should strive to get the necessary fat you need from healthier sources such as fresh milk, eggs, fatty fish, olive oil, avocados, and some tree nuts.

There are two types of dietary fats that are harmful and major contributors to high blood pressure, saturated fats and trans-fat. Most fats that have a high amount of saturated or trans-fat are solid at room temperature. These "solid fats" include beef fat, pork fat, vegetable shortening, margarine, and butter.

* Saturated Fat - This type of fat comes mainly from animal sources such as fatty meat and full-fat dairy products. Saturated fat raises total blood cholesterol and low-density (LDL) cholesterol which creates an increased risk for heart disease and stroke.

* Trans Fat - This type of fat is made from vegetable oils through a process called partial hydrogenation. Trans fats increase unhealthy LDL at a greater rate than saturated fat and it also lowers healthy high-density (HDL) cholesterol. Trans fats raise blood cholesterol more than any other food you can eat. It greatly increases your risk for heart disease. If you are concerned about having or getting high blood pressure you should immediately stop eating or using any product that contain trans fat. Read the nutrition labels of the foods you buy. The label can list 0 grams if the product has less than 0.5 grams. Look to see if it lists any hydrogenated or partially hydrogenated oils and if so do not buy it!

"There are two primary choices in life: to accept conditions as they exist, or accept the responsibility for changing them." - Denis Waitley

CHAPTER 5 ---
FINAL WORDS

"Knowledge is of no value unless you put it into practice." ~ Anton Chekhov

I truly hope that you have found this information useful. I personally know the anxiety of having a condition and not having enough information to ask the right questions when visiting a doctor. I extensively researched this information and, as described in several sections, applied many of the recommendations in my personal life. I have been able to achieve a marked blood pressure reduction by following the natural methods of blood pressure control presented in this book. I know it is not an easy task and the temptations to fall back into an unhealthy lifestyle are many. I do know that if you are trying, the changes get easier as they become more of a habit and you start feeling the effects of having a healthier lifestyle.

~~~~~~~~~~

Disclaimer:

As I said in the introduction, this book is not intended to be a replacement for professional medical care. The information in this book is based on the research and personal experiences of the author. Individuals who have been prescribed medication or placed on a special diet by their doctor or health care provider should talk with their doctor before making any dietary or exercise regimen changes suggested in this book.

The purpose of this book is educational only and is intended to give the reader a better understanding of the subject matter. By being more informed, you can improve your health and can help your doctor help you. I made every effort to give accurate and up to date information gained from my research but this book cannot be guaranteed to be free of factual error. You, the reader, are responsible for your own actions and agree to accept all risks before using any of the information presented in this book.

~~~~~~~~~~

"The doctor of the future will give no medicine, but will interest his patients in the care of the human frame, in diet and in the cause and prevention of disease." ~ Thomas Edison

~~~~~~~~~~

End

www.ingramcontent.com/pod-product-compliance
Lightning Source LLC
Chambersburg PA
CBHW062050280526
45788CB00003B/1177